Ultrasound and the Fallopian Tube

PROGRESS IN OBSTETRIC
AND GYNECOLOGICAL
SONOGRAPHY SERIES

SERIES EDITOR: ASIM KURJAK

Ultrasound and the Fallopian Tube

Edited by

ILAN E. TIMOR-TRITSCH and ASIM KURJAK

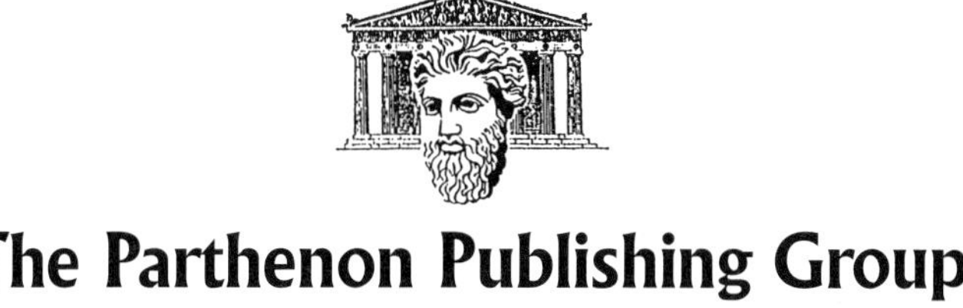

The Parthenon Publishing Group

International Publishers in Medicine, Science & Technology

NEW YORK   LONDON

British Library Cataloguing in Publication Data

Ultrasound and the fallopian tube. – (Progress in obstetric and gynecological sonography series)
1. Fallopian tube – Ultrasound imaging
I. Timor-Tritsch, Ilan E. II. Kurjak, Asim

618.1'2'07543

ISBN 1-85070-616-6

A Library of Congress Cataloging-in-Publication Data record is available from the Library of Congress

Published in the UK and Europe by
The Parthenon Publishing Group Limited
Casterton Hall, Carnforth
Lancs. LA6 2LA, UK

Published in North America by
The Parthenon Publishing Group Inc.
One Blue Hill Plaza
Pearl River
New York 10965, USA

Typesetting and reprographics by Laserprint, Macclesfield, Cheshire

Printed and bound by Butler & Tanner Ltd., Frome and London

Contents

List of principal contributors

Fatma A. Aleem
The Brookdale Hospital Medical Center
Department of Obstetrics and Gynecology
1335 Linden Boulevard
Brooklyn
NY 11212
USA

Fernando Bonilla-Musoles
Department of Obstetrics and Gynecology
Hospital Clínico Universitario
University of Valencia School of Medicine
Avenida Blasco Ibáñez 17
Valencia
Spain

Nathan Haratz-Rubinstein
Department of Obstetrics and Gynecology
Columbia Presbyterian Medical Center
630 West 168th Street
New York
New York 10032
USA

Debra S. Heller
College of Physicians and Surgeons
Columbia University, New York
630 West 168th Street
New York
NY 10032
USA

Ljiljana Kostović-Knežević
Department of Histology and Embriology
University of Zagreb School of Medicine
Salata 3
41000 Zagreb
Croatia

Sanya Kupešić
Department of Obstetrics and Gynecology
Medical School University of Zagreb
Sveti Duh 64
41000 Zagreb
Croatia

Asim Kurjak
Department of Obstetrics and Gynecology
Medical School University of Zagreb
Sveti Duh 64
41000 Zagreb
Croatia

Judi P. Lerner
Department of Obstetrics and Gynecology
Columbia Presbyterian Medical Center
622 West 168th Street PH Room 1212
New York
NY 10032
USA

Ana Monteagudo
Department of Obstetrics and Gynecology
Columbia Presbyterian Medical Center
630 West 168th Street
New York
NY 10032
USA

Ilan E. Timor-Tritsch
Department of Obstetrics and Gynecology
Columbia Presbyterian Medical Center
630 West 168th Street
New York
NY 10032
USA

Color plate 1 Transvaginal color Doppler image demonstrating a uterus with a decidual reaction (arrow). Left side, transverse view; right side, sagittal view

Color plate 2 Unilateral tubal twin pregnancy. Color Doppler imaging of the right Fallopian tube, revealing two independent gestational sacs without embryonic structures (arrows). Increased vascularity is present between both gestational sacs (arrow)

Color plate 3 Same patient as in Color plate 2. Color flow Doppler velocity waveform studies revealed low-resistance flows with resistance index 0.38 and pulsatility index 0.45 in the peritrophoblastic area

Color plate 4 Transvaginal color Doppler scan of a developing ectopic pregnancy

Color plate 5 Transvaginal color Doppler scan of a regressive ectopic pregnancy

Color plate 6 Trophoblastic color flow in an ectopic pregnancy

Color plate 7 Corpus luteum color flow in an ectopic pregnancy, showing the 'half-moon' pattern

Color plate 8 Unilocular cystic structure adherent to the uterus represents hydrosalpinx. Color and pulsed Doppler demonstrate characteristic blood flow pattern of uterine artery

Color plate 9 Same patient as in Color plate 8, magnified lower part of the hydrosalpinx. Note ovary at the edge of the cyst and blood flow signal of the uterine artery and internal iliac vein

Color plate 10 Color Doppler sonography of the small hydrosalpinx demonstrated as bilocular cyst. No vascularity of the cystic structure is demonstrated

Color plate 11 Multilocular cystic structure with irregular septa and intracystic echoes. Color Doppler shows blood flow located within the septa of the hydrosalpinx

Color plate 12 Same case as in Color plate 11; pulsed Doppler demonstrates moderate impedance to blood flow in the vessel located within the septa of the hydrosalpinx

Color plate 13 Tubular cystic structure can be misinterpreted as dilated vessel. Color Doppler shows absent blood flow within the tubular structure (arrow; tube), with diameter of 0.6 cm, confirming that this structure is not a dilated vessel

Color plate 14 Transvaginal color Doppler ultrasound of the Fallopian tube leiomyoma (arrows). The uterus (UT), the Fallopian tube (FT) and the fimbriated end (F) are clearly depicted

Color plate 15 Leiomyoma of the Fallopian tube (TL) reveals high-resistance flows, with RI 0.72 and PI 1.81

Color plate 16 Color flow imaging of the right tubal mass revealed 'hot' area of blood flow within the mass

Color plate 17 Doppler waveform analysis of the newly formed vessels in the tumor demonstrated low impedance to blood flow (RI = 0.35)

Color plate 18 Color flow imaging of the left adnexal mass reveals area of intensive ('hot') blood flow within the solid part of the mass. Note small papillary projection protruding into the tubal lumen

Color plate 19 The same patient as in Color plate 18. Doppler waveform analysis of the newly formed vessels in the tumor demonstrates low impedance to blood flow (RI = 0.38) and persistence of an arteriovenous shunt. Tubal malignancy was confirmed by histopathology

Color plate 20 Transvaginal color Doppler sonography demonstrated neovascularization in the solid part of the intraluminal growth of a Fallopian tube carcinoma. A sausage-shaped cystic mass with papillary projections extends from the inner surface

Color plate 21 Transabdominal color Doppler hystero-salpingography. Note color Doppler signals passing into the uterine cavity and both Fallopian tubes

Color plate 22 Bilateral proximal tubal occlusion demonstrating an abrupt cessation of saline flow and reflux of the fluid, shown in blue

Color plate 23 Transvaginal scan demonstrating two separate endometria in a case of septate uterus. Small myometrial vessels belonging to the uterine septum are easily detected by color Doppler. In such an obvious case there is no need for distention of the uterine cavity with fluid

Color plate 24 Long-axis transvaginal scan of the uterus after injection of the isotonic saline. Note hyperechoic avascular sessile structure representing endometrial polyp. On the left, small hypoechoic myoma distorts the adjacent endometrium. Color flow is obtained on its periphery

Color plate 25 The same patient as in Chapter 10, Figure 2. Regular peripheral vascularization is detected by color Doppler

Continued on page xv

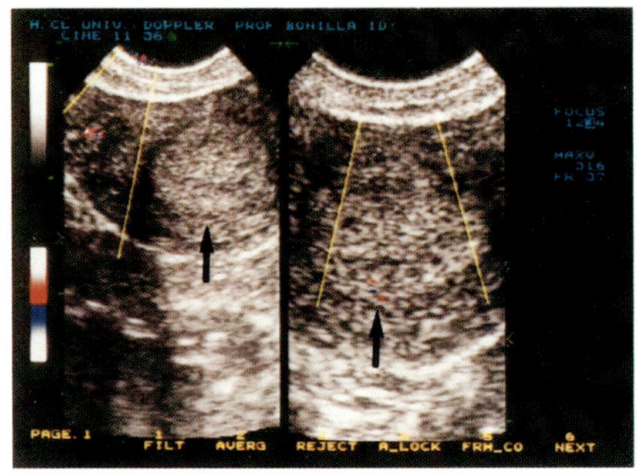

1

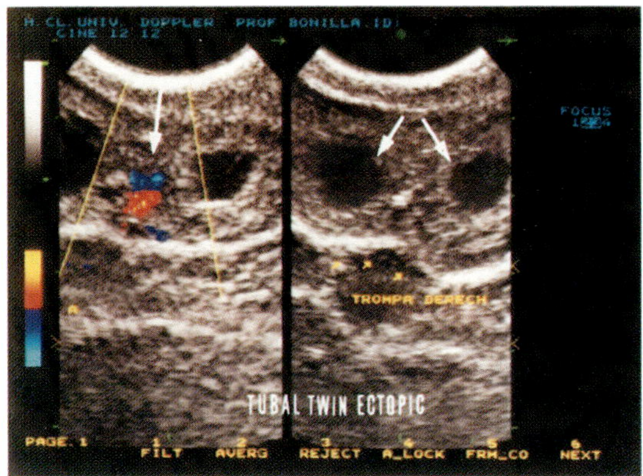

2

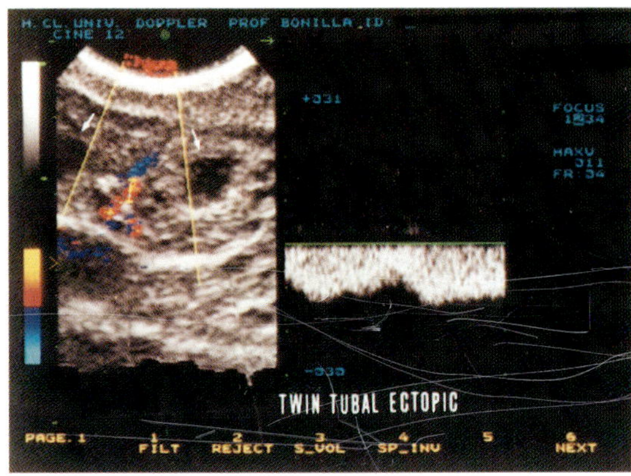

3

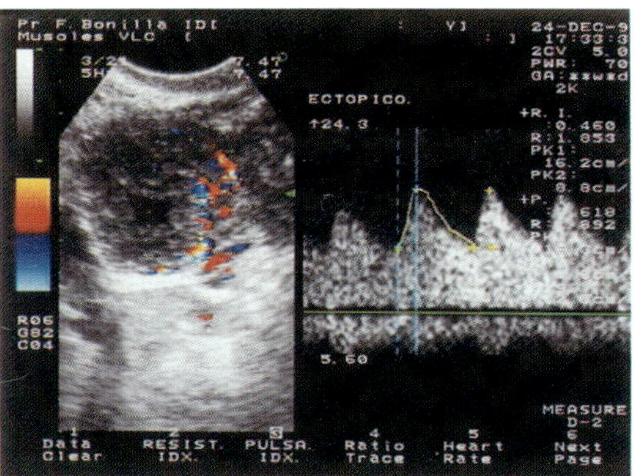

4

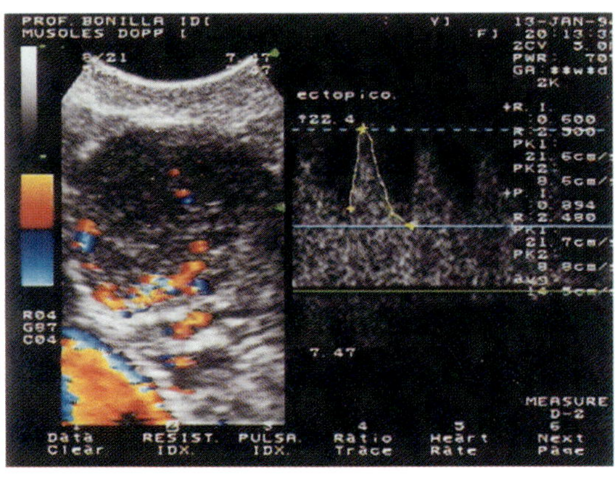

5

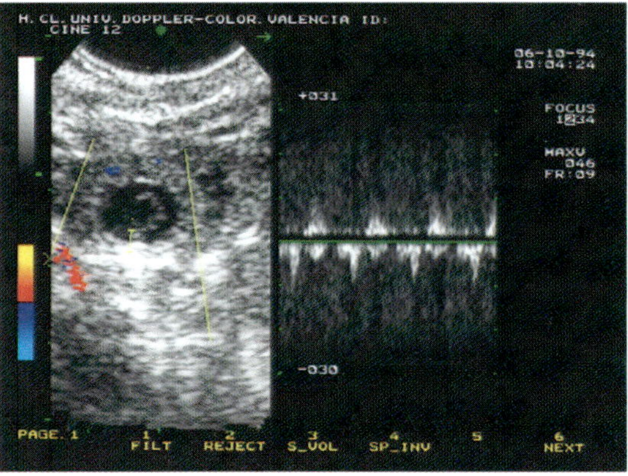

6

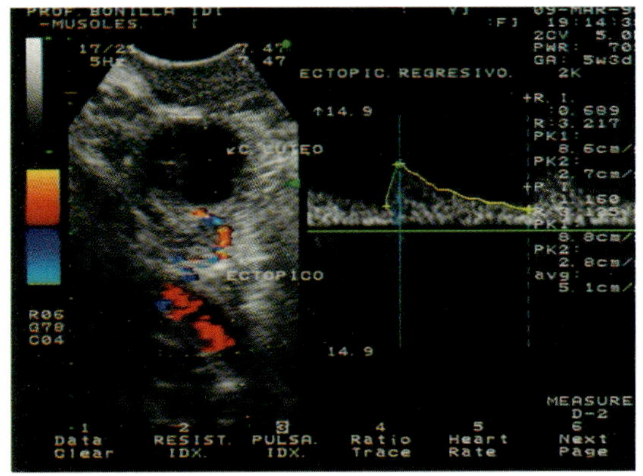

7

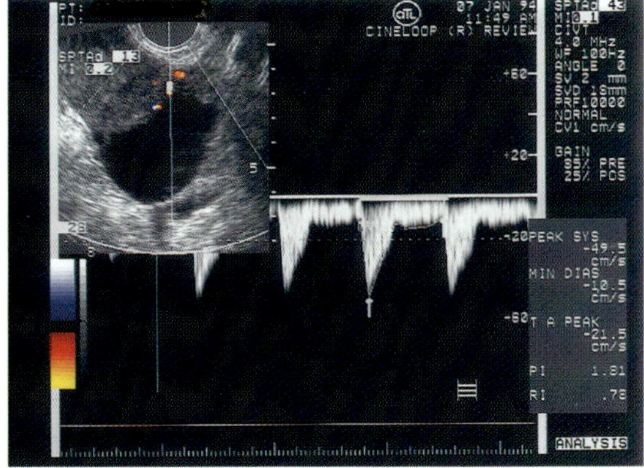

8

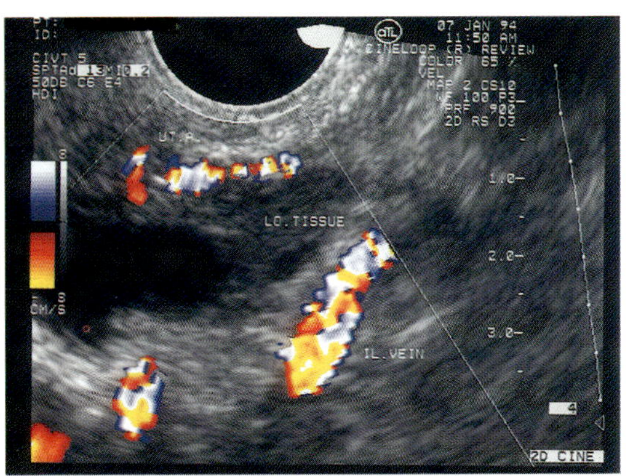

9

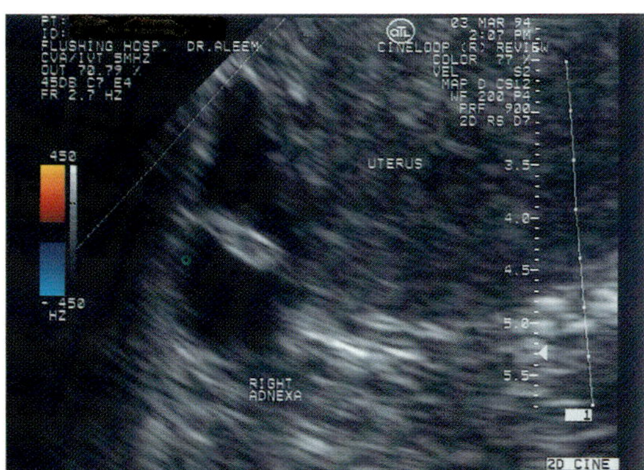

10

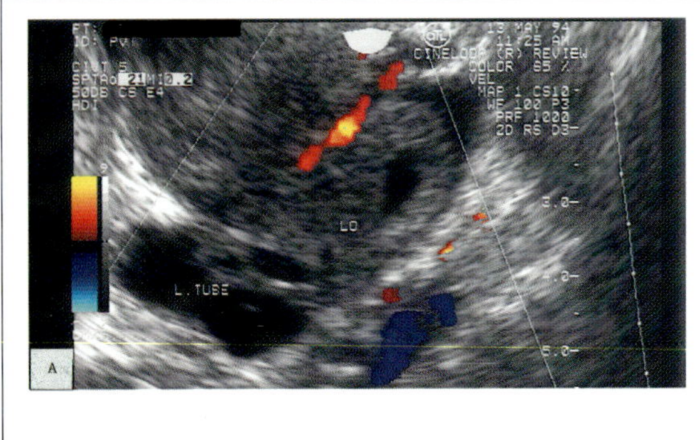

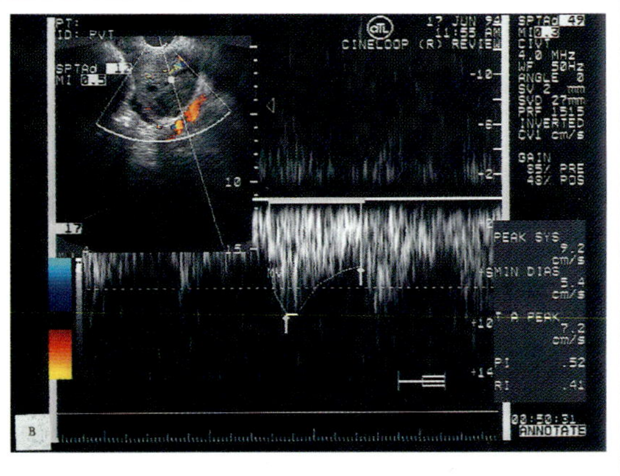

11

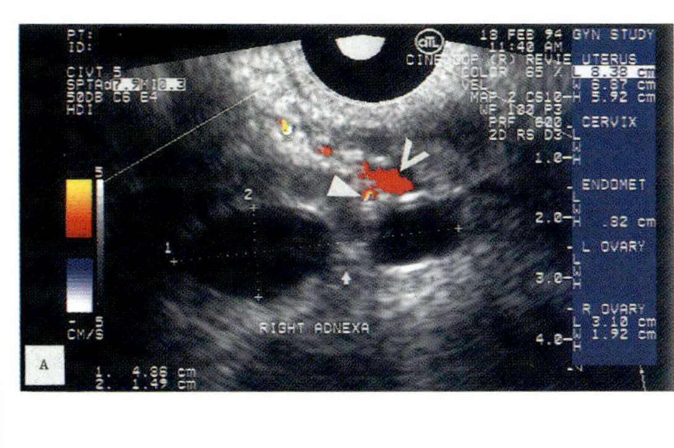

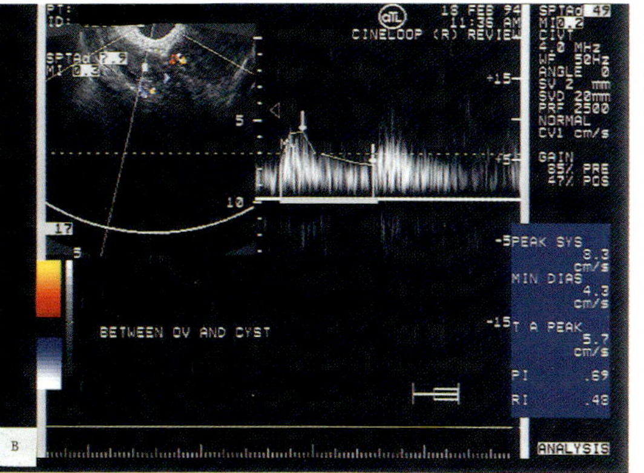

12

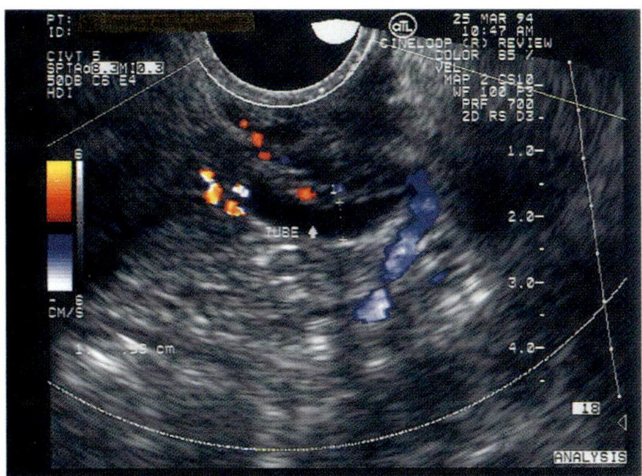

13

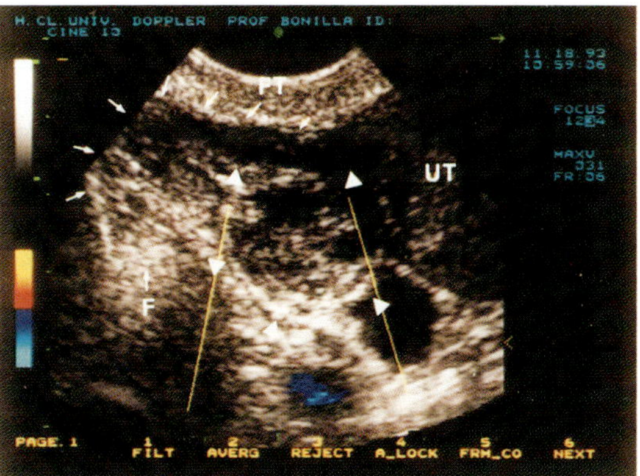

14

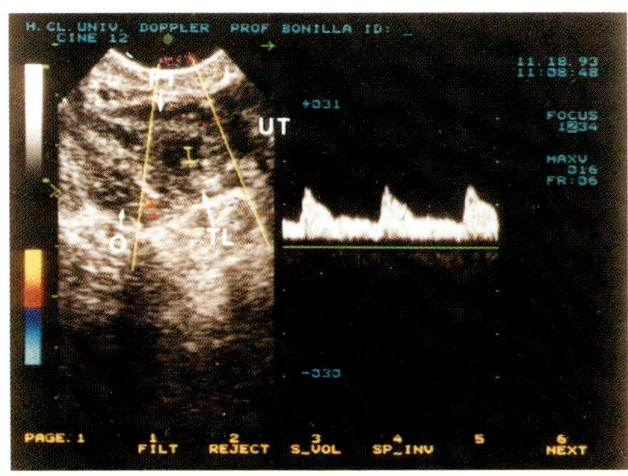

15

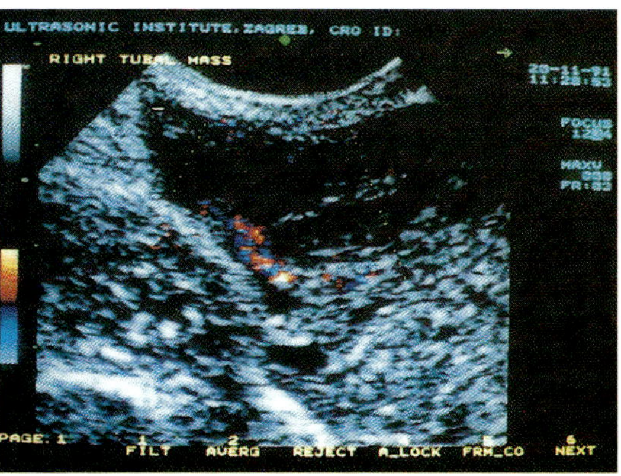

16

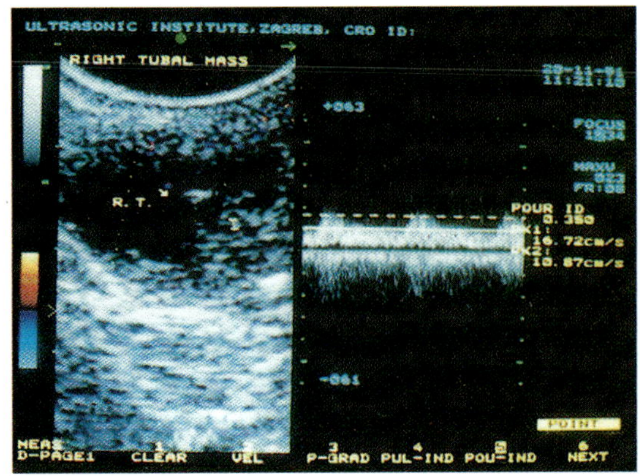

17

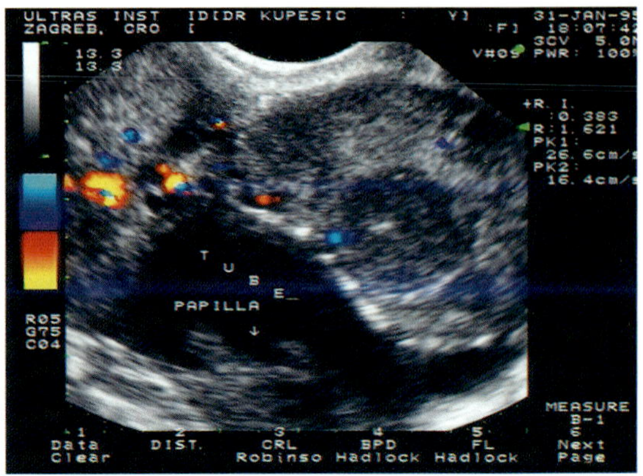

18

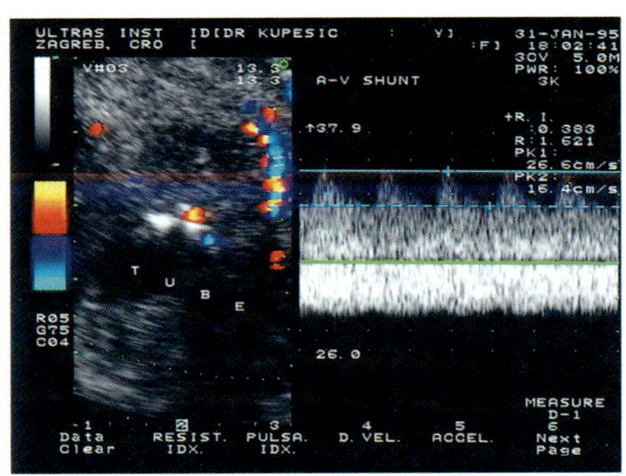

19

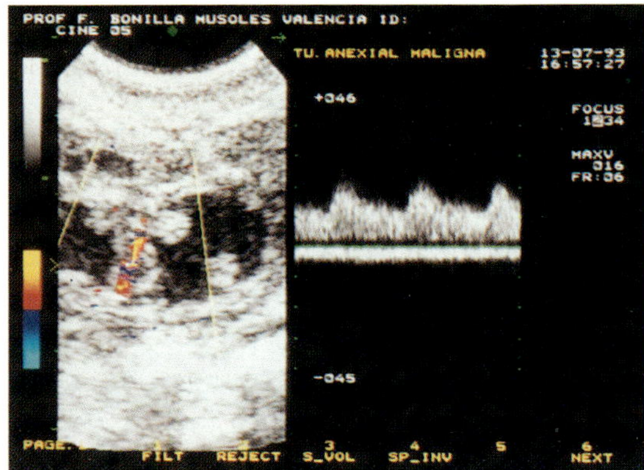

20

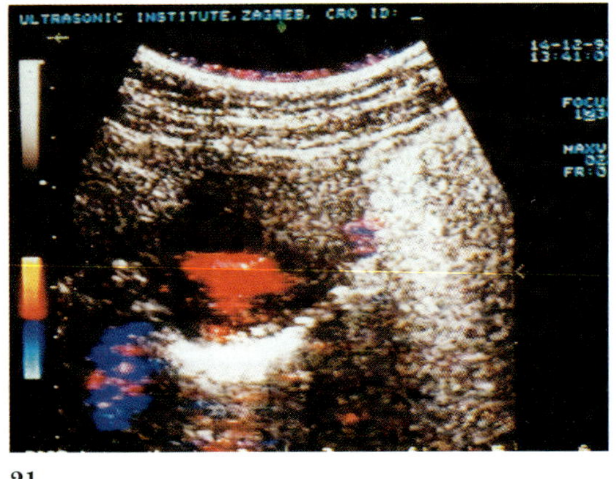

21

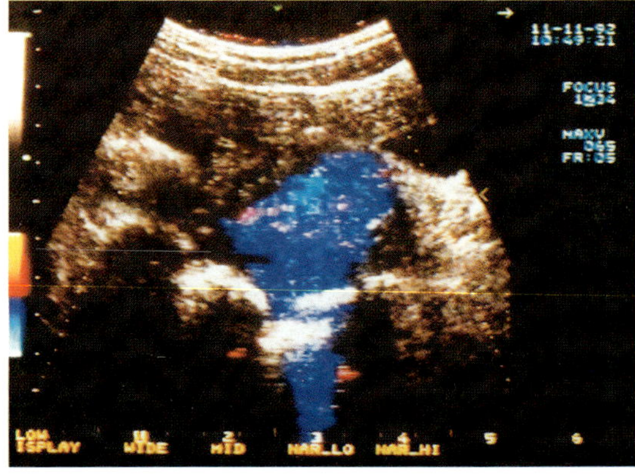

22

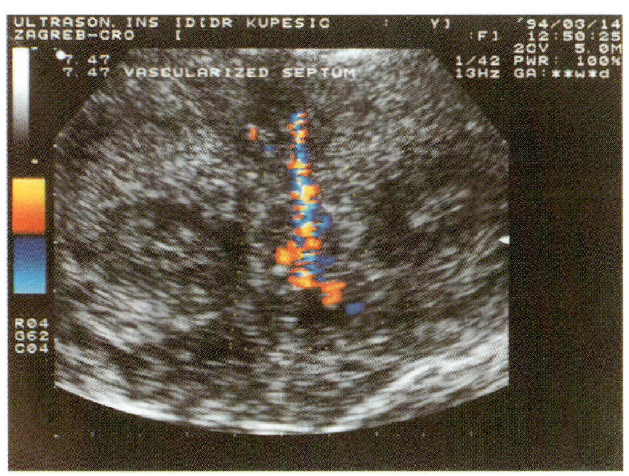

23

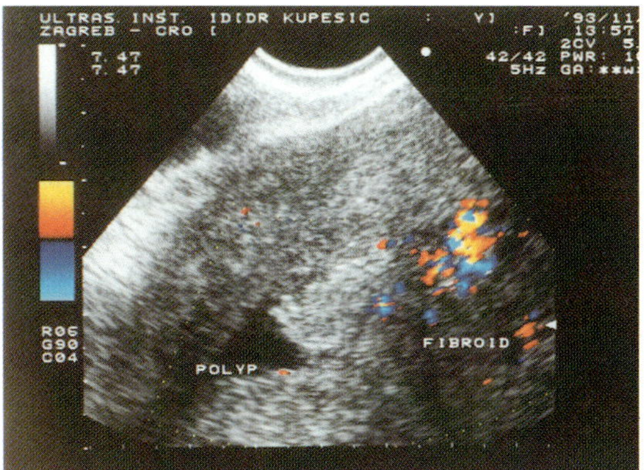

24

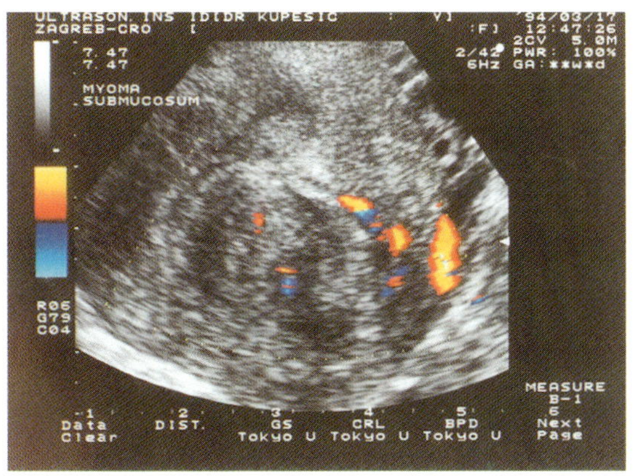

25

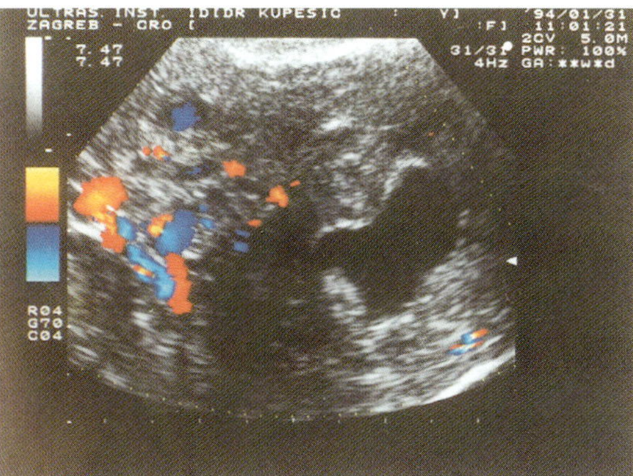

26

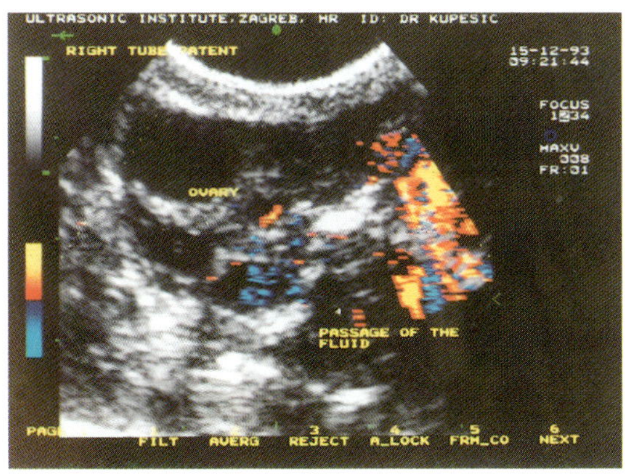

27

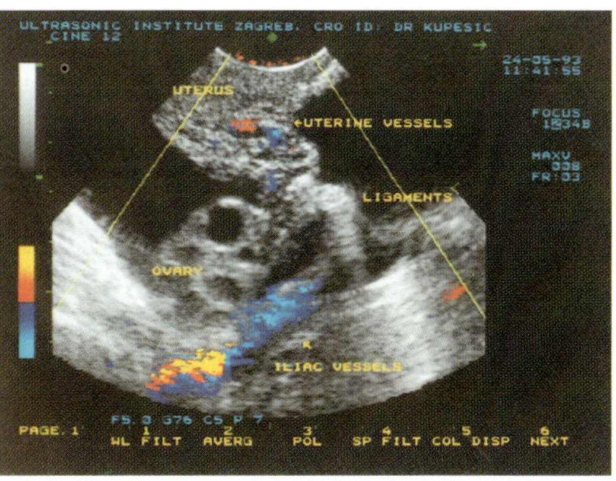

28

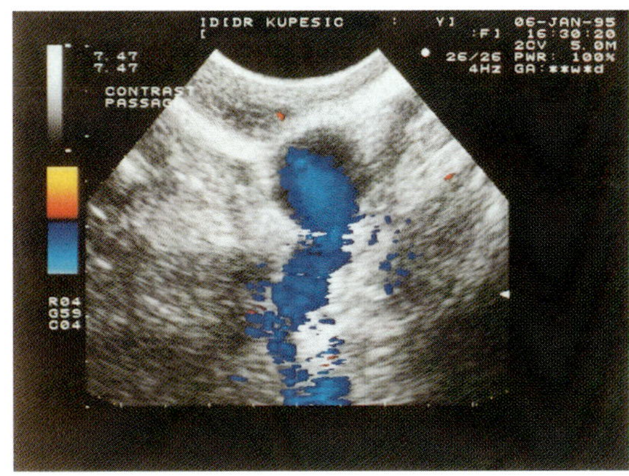

29

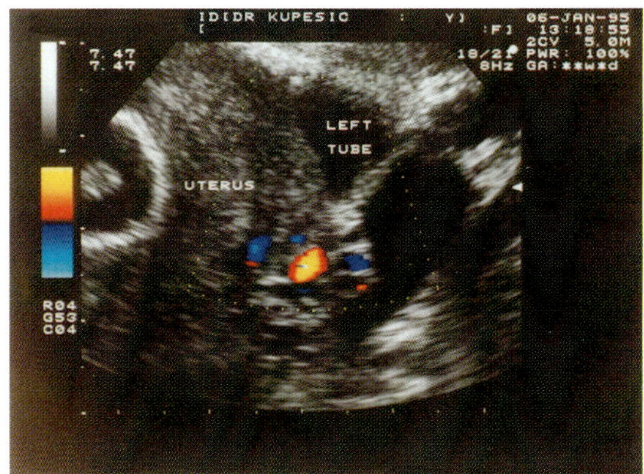

30

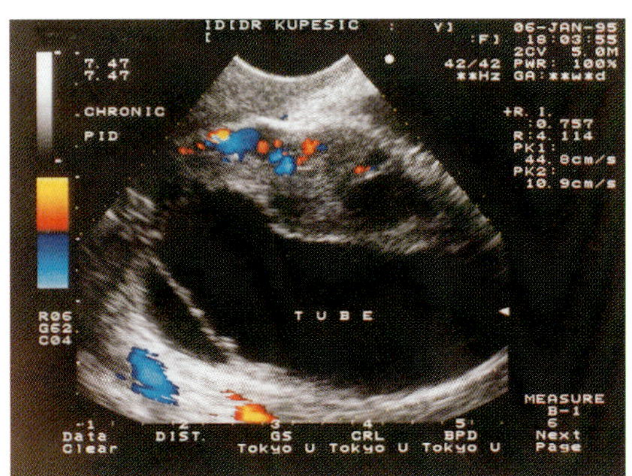

31

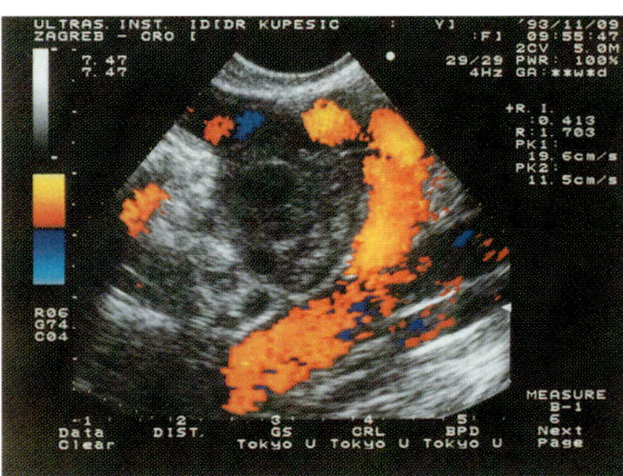

32

Continued from page viii

Color plate 26 Transvaginal scan of the uterus containing necrotic fibroid in an infertile patient. Instillation of the contrast media was done preoperatively in order to define if there is a sufficient distance between the capsule of myoma and the uterine cavity, and thus to estimate whether the uterine cavity needs to be opened

Color plate 27 Color Doppler hysterosalpingography. The color flow is saline passing through the right tube indicating normal tubal patency. Anechoic fluid is visualized in the cul-de-sac

Color plate 28 Color Doppler flow of saline passing into the posterior cul-de-sac. Note normal morphology of the left ovary and left tube floating in the fluid. Iliac vessels are clearly visible below the ovary

Color plate 29 Color signals passing through the left tube indicate normal tubal patency after color Doppler hysterosalpingography using selective tubal catheter

Color plate 30 Transvaginal color Doppler of the uterus and left adnexa. Note intrauterine catheter on the left. Color signals demonstrate inflow of the contrast into the left tube. The Fallopian tube is shown as a sausage-like septated structure caused by accumulation of the fluid proximal to the fimbriated end

Color plate 31 Iatrogenic hydrosalpinx after fluid injection in a patient with distal tubal occlusion. Color signals indicate passage of the contrast through the left cornual region. Note cyst-like structure representing dilated ampullar part of the left tube

Color plate 32 Color Doppler imaging answers the question whether the complex mass shown in Chapter 10, Figure 6 represents pelvic inflammatory disease or dilated veins. Pelvic congestion syndrome affecting peri-ovarian veins was proven by laparoscopy

Foreword

A little less than a decade ago, it would have seemed inconceivable to dedicate more than one chapter related to the subject of the Fallopian tube, leave alone an entire book. Transvaginal sonography has enabled a new look at this important organ, with its higher resolution and the ability to enhance it with color Doppler.

For those who seek a comprehensive text on the sonographic aspects of the Fallopian tube, starting with histopathological aspects and continuing through the normal sonographic appearance of the tube, as well as the intriguing picture of the inflamed salpinx, the appropriate chapters will be appreciated. The attempts to evaluate the tube through its vascularization, the relatively rare benign and malignant tumors as well as paratubal tumors are also discussed. Thanks to the efficient and early detection of ectopic pregnancies, this prevalent disease is now detected with a relative ease. The chapter discussing the ectopic gestation can serve as an aid to the practicing gynecologists to gain confidence in managing the patient suspected of this disease. A special chapter is dedicated to a relatively new procedure to test the patency of the Fallopian tube by ultrasonography.

We are confident that readers will find the text and the reference list useful in their search for support in rendering better patient care.

Ilan E. Timor-Tritsch
Asim Kurjak

The development and structure of the Fallopian tube   1

Lj. Kostović-Knežević and D. Grbeša

DEVELOPMENT OF THE HUMAN FALLOPIAN TUBE

Human embryos of both sexes exhibit the same developmental stage, when undifferentiated gonads are associated with mesonephric tubules. Two sets of gonad ducts, the Wolffian (mesonephric) and Müllerian (paramesonephric) ducts, develop and extend within the urogenital ridge. During organogenesis, one set of these ducts degenerates, while the other persists and differentiates into its derivatives[1]. Differentiation in the female includes the organization of the ovary and the Müllerian duct system, the regression of the Wolffian duct, and the differentiation of the external genitalia[2].

Embryonic period of development

The Wolffian ducts develop earlier than the Müllerian ducts[3]. During the 4th week, the mesonephric tubules develop and the Wolffian ducts begin to appear. During the 5th week, the primordia of the sex gonads arise[2].

After the sex of the gonads is distinguishable morphologically, the ducts begin to differentiate[4]. The Müllerian ducts appear during the 5th week, just about the time male differentiation begins[2,5,6]. They develop laterally to the gonads and Wolffian ducts and represent the primary structures from which the epithelium of the female genital organs will develop[7,8].

Embryos indicate the future Müllerian ducts by a groove in the thickened celomic epithelium of each urogenital ridge. The epithelial thickening elongates and forms a longitudinal groove. Its cranial end remains open into the celomic cavity as a funnel-like structure. More caudally, the lips of the groove close into a tube. The caudal tip of the invagination forms a solid bud of epithelium which gradually burrows in the mesenchyme[3]. The solid blind end of the Müllerian duct progressively grows caudally and courses lateral to the Wolffian duct. The Müllerian duct uses the Wolffian duct as a guiding structure[9]. Near the cloaca, the two urogenital ridges swing toward the midline and fuse into the genital cord[10].

In the 7th week, the Müllerian ducts are fully developed. They are simple, straight tubes lined with a single-layered epithelium which is enclosed by basal lamina. The Müllerian and Wolffian ducts run in parallel. The distance between them is short and it decreases in a caudal direction. The cross-sectional area of the Müllerian duct is approximately twice that of the Wolffian duct (widest diameters are 90 µm and 55 µm, respectively). This difference also diminishes during the 7th and the 8th weeks. The lumen of the Müllerian duct is narrow and the cells form a columnar epithelium. At this stage of development, the mesenchymal cells around the Müllerian duct differentiate in the periductal stroma. Light and electron microscopic studies show two types of mesenchymal cells: spindle-shaped, fusiform or stellate cells with a dense cytoplasm (dark cells) and epitheloid cells with ovoid nuclei and a less intensively stained cytoplasm (light cells)[11].

Sexual differentiation of the reproductive tract is dependent on the endocrine secretion of fetal testes. Two testicular hormones play an important role[12]. The onset of testicular differentiation may be at postgestational day 42. At about day 56, the Sertoli cells in the fetal testes begin to secrete Müllerian inhibiting substance (MIS), a glycoprotein also known as anti-Müllerian hormone (AMH). MIS is one of the earliest products of the fetal testis. If it is secreted in sufficient amounts, it

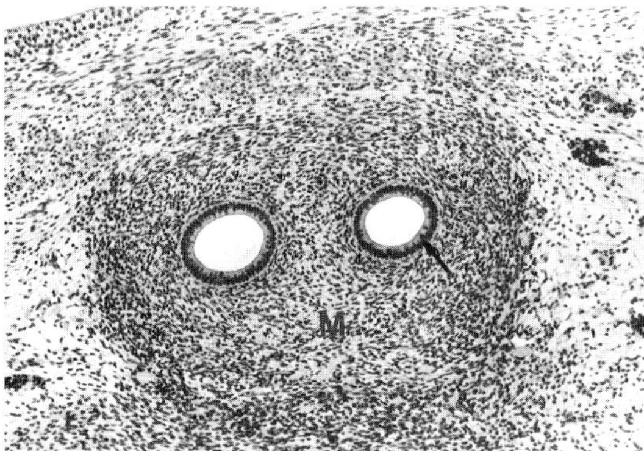

Figure 1 The Müllerian ducts in 8-week-old human embryo. The cells form a columnar epithelium (arrow). The mesenchymal cells (M) differentiate in the periductal stroma ($\times$ 189)

inhibits development of the Müllerian duct and initiates its regression in male fetuses[13]. In normal development, MIS is expressed in the gonads of both sexes but with distinct temporal patterns[14]. MIS is produced by fetal and adult testes, and by granulosa cells of the postnatal ovary. Steroidal androgens, secreted by fetal testes, maintain the mesonephric tubules and Wolffian ducts, stimulate their morphogenesis and development of the male genital organs. The developing Müllerian ducts are sensitive to MIS during a specific period: exposure before or after this period has no effect on Müllerian duct regression[5]. Organ culture experiments of embryonic human gonads indicate that the developing Müllerian ducts are sensitive to MIS from approximately the 6th to the 8th or the 9th week of gestation[15–17]. After this time, the Müllerian ducts become insensitive to MIS. Female sexual development does not depend on the presence of ovaries or on any direct hormonal stimulus of gonadal origin[5, 7, 18]. The fetal ovary does not secrete a hormone in sufficient amounts to have any influence and the development of the female duct system is self-differentiating and independent of such control[7]. In the absence of fetal testes, Wolffian ducts and mesonephric tubules degenerate due to a lack of stimulation from androgens[1, 4]. In the absence of MIS, the Müllerian duct persists and continues to grow in a caudo-medial direction (Figure 1).

During the 8th week, stromal cells form a more compact stratum of concentrically arranged layers around the Müllerian duct[11].

Early fetal period of development

During the 9th week, the Müllerian duct progressively elongates, its blind tip reaches the pelvic area and the duct crosses in front of the Wolffian duct to its medial side. In the 9th week, the stroma develops fully. Light and dark cells form a compact layer encircling the epithelial duct[11]. The thickness of this stratum varies between 20 and 30 µm. Two or three layers of light cells form the inner stromal sheet; four or five layers of dark cells form the outer stromal sheet and continue into the loose mesenchymal tissue. The light cells completely envelope the duct and form a very compact tissue. Most cells of outer sheet are flat and form concentric lamellae. Due to the small amount of cytoplasm and the flat nuclei, the peripheral zone of the periductal stroma is characterized by a high degree of compactness. The amount of extracellular space increases and contains collagen fibrils. The ductal cells change into a regular low columnar epithelium.

In the 10th week, the Müllerian ducts fuse in the midline in a Y-shape and form the uterovaginal canal (primordia of the body and the cervix of the uterus and the vagina)[19]. At this time, the uterovaginal canal is straight and lined by immature columnar (Müllerian) epithelium[5]. When the urogenital ridges are crowded laterally by the enlarging suprarenal glands and permanent kidneys, the Müllerian ducts participate in this displacement. The part of the Müllerian duct between the ovary and uterovaginal canal remains slender and forms the oviduct[20]. Near its cranial end, the ostium develops. The tip of the duct may persist as a vesicular appendage attached to the oviduct, a hydatid of Morgagni[7, 21].

At early stages of differentiation, the Müllerian ducts are lined with a single-layered epithelium. During normal organogenesis, the mesenchyme induces and specifies epithelial morphogenesis and cytodifferentiation[22]. The mesenchymal cells induce differentiation of embryonic Müllerian epithelium into a simple columnar epithelium of the oviduct and uterus[1, 23, 24].

As the Müllerian ducts grow, the epithelium becomes taller, with the nuclei situated in the basal part of cells. Parallel to the epithelial growth, mesenchymal cells are arranged in concentric layers around the ducts. Further differentiation of the genital ducts depends on mesenchymal–epithelial interaction. The mesenchyme is the target and mediator of morphogenic action by sex hormones[22,25]. Hormonal sensitivity in morphogenic processes is a result of hormone–receptor activity within mesenchyme. The balance of estrogen to androgen in the circulation may be critical in modulating MIS activity[5]. Analysis of developing estrogen target organs indicates hormone–receptor activity within mesenchymal cells. Receptors for estrogen are localized in mesenchymal cells surrounding the Müllerian duct, Wolffian duct and urogenital sinus of rat or mouse offspring[12,26]. These cells induce differentiation of embryonic Müllerian epithelium into a simple columnar epithelium lining the oviduct and uterus[1,23,24].

The early differentiating oviduct can be distinguished from the uterus by its coiling and smaller diameter. A muscular layer develops around the oviductal tube. The oviductal epithelium invaginates and folds. The epithelial cells may either develop cilia or later become secretory. The oviduct differentiates into three segments: the infundibulum, the ampulla and the isthmus. In humans, most of these developmental steps occur during the midgestational period. The junction between oviduct and uterus becomes clearly distinguishable at an early stage by the abrupt increase in uterine diameter[25].

Between the 8th and 10th week, the Müllerian duct shows a moderate decrease of its diameter[11]. In the upper part of the Müllerian duct, the outer stromal sheet consists mainly of dark, spindle-shaped cells. The inner sheet does not exhibit compact arrangement of the light, epitheloid cells.

During the 10–12th weeks, the number of light cells decreases but the diameter of the duct and periductal stroma remains constant.

The epithelial cells lining the human fetal Fallopian tube may be classified into four main types:

(1) Microvillous;

(2) Fully ciliated;

(3) Microvillous and ciliated; and

(4) Possessing a centrally located single cilium[8].

The prenatal differentiation of the epithelial cells lining the oviduct has been studied in various mammals[27,28]. Differentiation of the ciliated cells of the mammalian oviduct usually begins earlier than that of the secretory cells.

At the 12th week of gestation, the Fallopian tube has a single-layer columnar epithelium without ciliated cells. The columnar cells possess many microvilli protruding into the slit-like lumen. A solitary cilium is occasionally present. The epithelium is demarcated from the underlying stroma by a basal lamina[29].

After the 12th week, the duct is surrounded by a coat of spindle-shaped cells. The intact basal lamina remains preserved and separates the stroma from the duct. Along the basal lamina, bundles of collagen fibers differentiate. The diameter of the upper portion of the Müllerian duct increases and the columnar cells elongate. The epithelium grows in height and the lumen expands[11].

From the 14th week of development, the oviductal mucosa are arranged in folds. They consist of an epithelial layer and stroma derived from the surrounding mesenchyme. The epithelium consists of a single layer of cuboidal or columnar cells with ovoidal or elongated nuclei. The monolayered epithelium appears 'pseudostratified'. The light cells (a polyhedral shape, clear cytoplasm and a spheroidal, vesicular nucleus with dispersed chromatin) are less numerous and intermingled with the dark cells (taller, cuboidal or columnar cells with elongated nucleus and a large nucleolus). The luminal side of the oviductal epithelial cells projects cilia and/or microvilli. Fimbriae are not yet well developed. The inner oviductal surface develops infoldings and furrows. At this stage of development, most epithelial cells of the human fetal oviduct are microvillous cells. Ciliated cells are interspersed among them[8].

The muscular and connective tissues of the oviduct begin to develop from mesenchyme during the 3rd month (Figure 2). By midpregnancy, they have a characteristic arrangement. The differentiation of the ampullar portion of the oviduct with its complex folds occurs mostly in the last third of gestation[3].

Between the 15th and the 18th week, the cytoplasm organelles of the oviductal epithelial cells

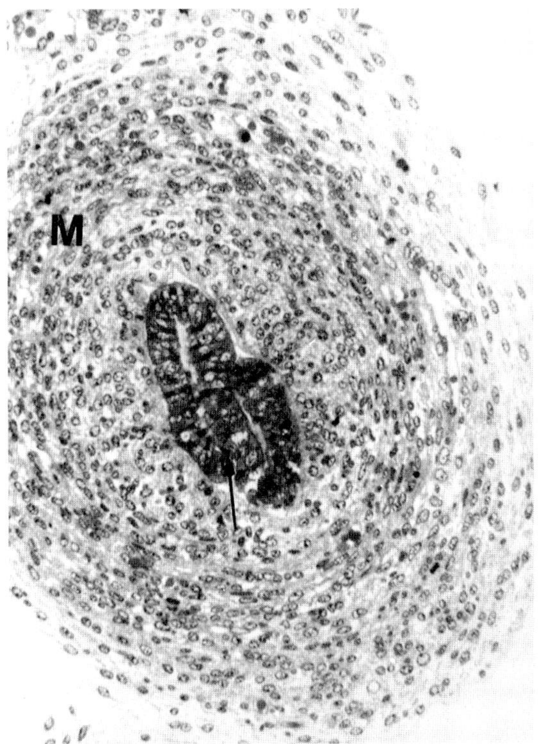

Figure 2 The semithin (1 µm thick) cross-section of the Fallopian tube in the 17th week of human development. The monolayered epithelium appears 'pseudostratified' (arrow). The mesenchyme (M) (× 173)

become better developed. They include mitochondria, rough endoplasmic reticula, free ribosomes, Golgi complexes and glycogen particles. Until the 18th week, fully ciliated cells are not identified, although cells possessing a solitary cilium are occasionally present. The ultrastructure of oviductal cells prior to the 18th week of development represents the indifferent stage of development of Müllerian epithelial cells[29].

At the 18th week, the proximal oviductal segment develops fimbriae. Ciliated cells are settled among the microvillous cells and they also develop at the uterotubal junction[8].

At the 20th week, the mucosal folds increase. The ampulla shows either few or no ciliated cells. Ciliogenesis is still present but ciliated elements progressively decrease in the infundibulo-ampullary zone. In the ampulla, the cells with a single cilium are the most abundant[8]. Some investigators confuse the undifferentiated cell having a single cilium with the ciliated cell having numerous cilia. This is one reason why the data of many investigators do not always agree. The cells having a single cilium are considered to be quite different from the ciliated cells. A solitary or single cilium, also termed rudimentary cilium or temporary cilium, was observed on the undifferentiated cells of the fetal oviduct. Although the cells having a solitary cilium tend to decrease in number with age, this structure sometimes persists in a fully differentiated secretory cell[30]. Occasional ciliated cells appear at the 20th week. They have cilia with a 9 + 2 microtubular structure. The cilia are a little shorter and not so strong and vigorous as seen in the tubes of fertile women[31]. Glycogen particles identified during the 18th week are not present at this stage. Several membrane-bound granules resembling lysosomes occur in the supranuclear region of ciliated cells[29]. The microvillous cells have club-shaped microvilli on their luminal surface. Microvilli suggest exchange of substances through the cell membrane at this early stage of development[31].

The fibromuscular layer is well developed. In 18–21-week-old human fetal oviduct, the vasculature differs from the vascular architecture of the oviduct in adult. The vasculature of fetal oviduct is supplied by anastomosing arterial branches of the uterine and ovarian arteries in the mesosalpinx with large veins. Larger arteries and veins, 70–100 µm in diameter, are located in the subserosal layer[32].

The intramural vasculature of the muscular layer and mucosal folds has not been differentiated into the arterial and venous system. It consists of capillary and sinusoidal networks. This lack of development reflects the functional immaturity of the oviduct.

In the infundibular region, longitudinal arteries and veins communicate with a dense mucosal network of capillaries.

The mucosal folds are well developed in the ampulla and contain only capillary vessels but without arteriole, venule stem typical of the mucosal fold in the mature oviduct. The mucosal capillaries have uneven contours and a diameter from 10 to 25 µm. In the outer surface of the ampulla, larger arteries give off arteriolar branches which supply the mucosal vasculature. They are accompanied by semicircular venules

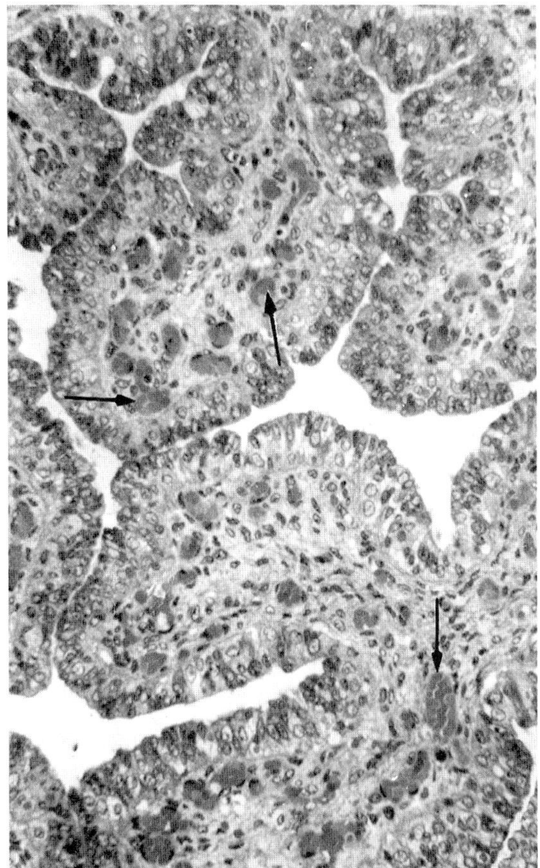

Figure 3 The semithin (1 μm thick) cross-section of the Fallopian tube in the 27th week of human development. The mucosal folds contain capillaries (arrows) (× 177)

draining the capillary bed and joining larger veins on the external surface of the oviduct. Such semicircular vessels are also observed in the mature oviduct. Semicircular arterioles do not show the spiralization that occurs in the mature oviduct[32].

The isthmic segment and its transition into the uterine wall are characterized by a prominent subserosal venous plexus composed of large vessels[32].

At 20–22 weeks, epithelial non-ciliated cells have well-developed organelles but do not contain lysosomes. The apical portion of the cytoplasm often protrudes toward the lumen but secretory granules are missing[29].

The secretory cells of the fetal oviductal epithelium in humans develop at midgestation[33]. The initial signals of differentiation of the secretory cells are enlargement of the Golgi complex and an increase of elements of rough endoplasmic reticulum. Increase in size and activity of these organelles occurs preliminary to the formation of secretory granules in these cells[30].

At the 22nd week of development, the oviductal epithelium shows pseudostratification. The epithelium is composed of light and dark cells, separated from the stroma by a basal lamina. Light cells are either microvillous, ciliogenic or fully ciliated. The luminal surfaces exhibit microvilli or cilia at varous developmental stages. The dark cells possess smooth luminal surfaces and elongated nuclei with condensed chromatin. Dark cells show features of degeneration and undergo apoptosis. The degenerate elements in the lumen of the human fetal tube are the morphological expression of a continuous epithelial remodelling during its differentiation. On the surface of the fimbriae, ciliated cells are increased in number. The ciliation is reduced in the direction of the uterus. The ciliated cells in the cranial oviductal segments are distributed in reverse ratio to the microvillous cells[8]. The microvillous cells possessing a single cilium are the more abundant elements. In the uterotubal junction, the number of ciliated cells increases again.

At the 24th week, the well-developed fimbriae consist of longitudinal infoldings separated by deep furrows (Figure 3).

Late fetal period of development

At the 31st week, the fetal oviductal mucosa seems hypertrophic. The fimbriae are indented and raised. The mucosal folds of the ampulla are covered by microvillous cells with secretory activity of apocrine type[8]. Accumulations of glycogen particles are again present in the cytoplasm of the epithelial cells. The ciliated cells are only sporadically present among non-ciliated cells[29].

The distribution of ciliated cells in late fetal oviduct is similar to that in the fimbriae and ampulla of adult humans[8]. Cell differentiation, their distribution in various segments of human fetal oviduct and secretory activity are dependent upon hormones circulating in the fetal blood vessels.

At the 40th week, the villous epithelial foldings resemble the epithelium of the adult (Figure 4). Ciliated cells are fully developed and large in

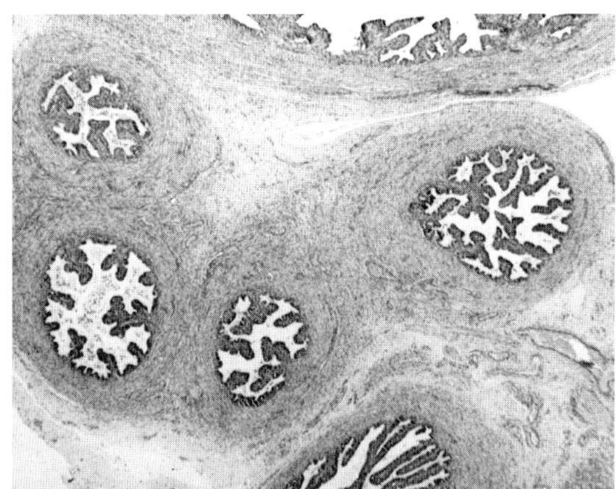

Figure 4   The cross-sections of the Fallopian tube in the 38th week of human development. The changes in the luminal diameter and the complexity of the mucosal folds are seen (× 20)

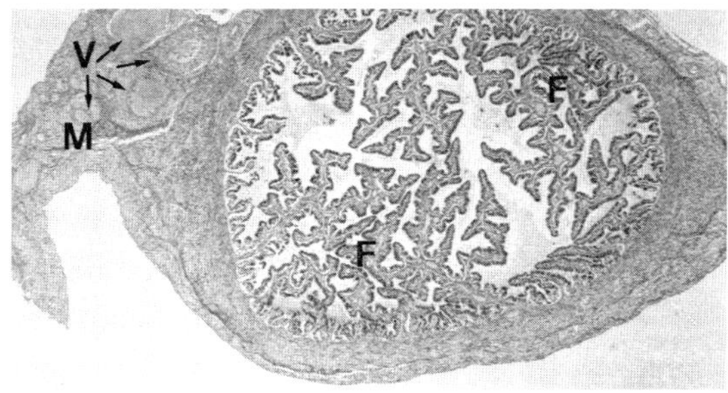

Figure 5   Transverse section of the ampullar part of the Fallopian tube. The mesosalpinx (M) with blood vessels (V) and numerous folds of the mucosa (F) are shown (×14)

number. They have prominent lysosomal granules in the supranuclear region. Most have multi-lamellar structures. Non-ciliated cells tend to protrude into the lumen but they are without secretory granules. The phenomenon of glycogen accumulation and disappearance probably relates to the differentiation of ciliated cells in oviductal epithelium. In the human fetus, two episodes of ciliogenesis appear, one at midgestation and the other at term[29].

The oviductal epithelial cells are already differentiated into both ciliated cells and secretory cells in the newborn human[34–36]. This epithelium resembles that of the adult except for the absence of cyclic changes and the presence of a smaller number of ciliated cells[30].

The trumpet-like cranial ends of the young Fallopian tube finally lie opposite the fourth lumbar vertebra, 13 segments below their level of origin[10].

STRUCTURE OF THE FALLOPIAN TUBE

The oviducts extend bilaterally from the uterus to the region of the ovary. In the sexually mature human female, they are 7–12 cm in length. They are suspended by a rather loose mesentery, the mesosalpinx, a derivative of the broad ligament (Figure 5).

The oviducts can be divided into four linear segments distinguishable by gross examination and by studying transverse sections taken at different levels. The first segment, the intramural portion (pars interstitialis) is situated in the interior of the uterine wall. The second segment (isthmus) is formed by the portion of the tube adjacent to the uterus. The third (ampulla) is the expanded segment which comprises about half the oviductal length. The fourth segment, the funnel-shaped abdominal opening (infundibulum) is situated near the ovary. The free margin of the infundibulum is extensively folded and fluted, giving it a tentacle-like appearance. These folds are called fimbriae.

The blood supply of the uterine tube comes from the vascular arch formed by anastomosis of the ovarian and uterine arteries, from which branches pass through the mesosalpinx to reach the muscular wall. Venous drainage is arranged in a similar vascular arch provided through the ovarian and uterine venous plexus (Figure 5).

Nerves supplying the uterine tube arrive in the part along the uterovaginal plexus and in the part accompanying the ovarian vessels.

Histological organization

The wall of the oviduct is composed of three layers: a mucosa, a muscular layer and an external serosa composed of visceral peritoneum.

The mucosa comprises longitudinally oriented primary and smaller secondary folds. The mucosa in the ampulla is thick and forms numerous branched folds (Figure 6). In the isthmus the longitudinal folds are short and less highly

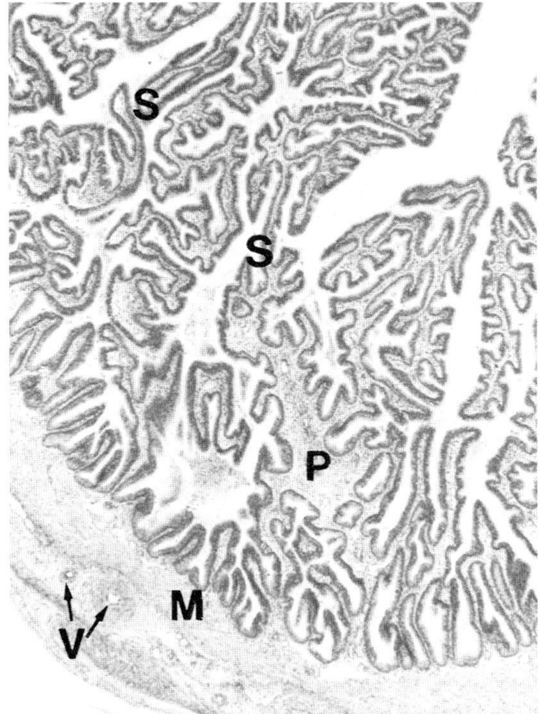

Figure 6 Transverse section of the ampullar wall. Primary (P) and secondary (S) branching folds of the mucosa and muscular layer (M) with blood vessels (V) are shown ($\times$ 173)

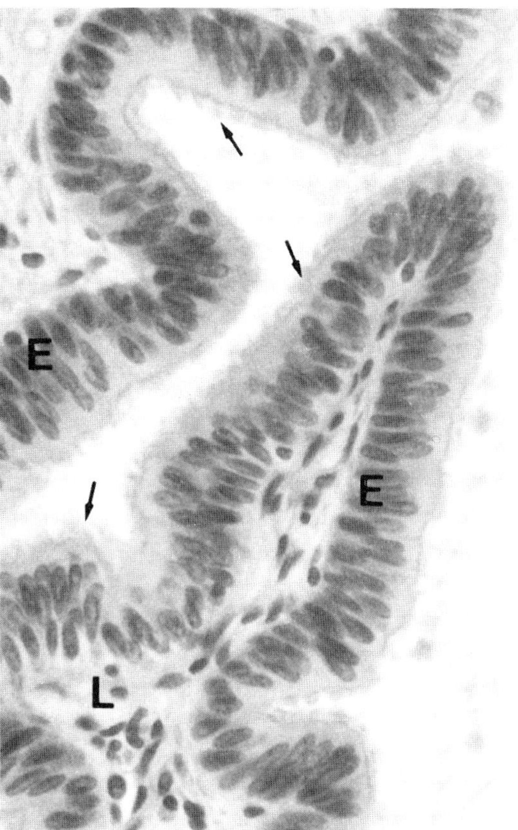

Figure 7 The surface columnar epithelium lining the mucosa (E). Some of them have numerous cilia (arrows). Lamina propria (L) is composed of loose connective tissue ($\times$ 316)

Histophysiology of the surface epithelium

branched. In the interstitial part they are reduced to the ridges.

The epithelium of the mucosa is simple columnar, consisting of several morphologically and functionally different kinds of cells.

The lamina propria of the mucosa is composed of loose connective tissue (Figures 6 and 7). There are reticular fibers and numerous cells. The fixed cells here seem to have the same developmental potential as those in the stroma of the uterus. In cases of abnormal nidation of an embryo, the cells of the lamina propria react like the endometrium, forming numerous decidual cells. Lamina propria contains abundant blood and lymph vessels of small diameter.

The next layer is the muscularis. It consists of an inner circular or spiral and an outer longitudinal layer of smooth muscle cells (Figure 6). Toward the uterus, the muscularis increases in thickness.

The outer, peritoneal, layer has a serosal structure (connective tissue and mesothelium).

The epithelium lining the mucosa is simple columnar and contains several types of cells (Figure 7). The morphology of the tubal epithelium based on classical histological techniques[34,37] reveals three principal types of the surface epithelium: ciliated, non-ciliated, or secretory, and 'peg' cells.

The use of transmission and scanning electron microscopic techniques reveals two types of cells: ciliated and secretory[38–40]. The 'peg' cells are merely one stage in the cyclic alterations of the secretory cells resulting from extrusion of the cytoplasm.

The first type of epithelial cells consists of those with numerous specialized structures called cilia on their free surface. Cilia are motile cell processes arranged in rows with microvilli between them. They are 7–10 µm long and 0.2 µm in diameter and easily resolved with the light microscope. Under the electron microscope, cilia are found to have a core structure, called the axoneme, consisting of longitudinal microtubules that have a constant number. Each cilium consists of two central and nine peripheral pairs of microtubules composed of structural proteins α and β tubulin. Each tubule pair has an inner and an outer cross-arm composed of high-molecular weight proteins known as dyneins. Cilia attach specifically to the structures in the apical region of the cell, called basal bodies[41]. From the basal bodies, cilia arise in the oviduct in response to hormonal stimulation. The specific movements characteristic of cilia, known as beating, involve a complex sliding of microtubules within each cilium. The beating of cilia is co-ordinated within each cell and at the same time within a group of several cells, resulting in spreading waves of motion which propagate the transport of oocytes through the ampulla to the ampullo-isthmic junction[41]. Ciliated cells are most densely distributed on the fimbria in the ampulla and are relatively sparsely distributed in the isthmus[42, 43].

Ultrastructural studies reveal that secretory cells have numerous small vesicles evident in the tip; these represent intracellular accumulation and storage of their secretory products. The cytoplasm also contains organelles involved in the synthetic activities of the cell: tubular profiles of granular endoplasmic reticulum in the basal cytoplasm, a prominent supranuclear Golgi region and tubular mitochondria[40].

Cyclic changes in the oviduct epithelium

During the menstrual cycle, both secretory and ciliated cells undergo morphological changes.

Some authors have studied qualitative and quantitative structural and ultrastructural characteristics of the tubal epithelium during reproductive life[31, 40, 42, 44–46].

The ciliation, increase of epithelial height and increased mitotic activity occur during the follicular phase, whereas deciliation, decrease of epithelial height and loss of mitotic activitiy coincide with the luteal phase and with elevated levels of serum progesterone. Maximal ciliation is attained around the time of ovulation. The maximum height of cells before ovulation coincides with the maximum activity of the secretory cells. That estrogen is important in ciliogenesis, cell height and mitotic activity may be demonstrated in oviduct from postmenopausal patients. After the menopause, the epithelium is low cuboidal and there are few ciliated cells[31, 45–47]. After long-term estrogen therapy, a ciliated epithelium is renewed, and is similar to that in women of reproductive age[46–49].

Immunohistochemical studies using qualitative and quantitative receptor assays have found the localization and distribution of estrogen and progesterone receptors in the epithelial and stromal cells in the Fallopian tube[50–55]. The results of immunohistochemical studies show that, in the Fallopian tube, epithelial and stromal estrogen receptors increase in the follicular phase to a peak at midcycle and then decline in the luteal phase. The fimbrial end demonstrates an opposite pattern of immunostaining to other segments of the tube. Progesterone receptor immunostaining is more intense than that for estrogen receptors in the follicular phase. The results for the fimbrial epithelium are a mirror image to the other regions of the tube[55]. These differences in the steroid receptor content may reflect the changing and different functional roles of these regions and may have important implications for human reproduction.

References

1. Cunha, G.R. (1976). Epithelial–stromal interactions in development of the urogenital tract. *Int. Rev. Cytol.*, **47**, 137–94
2. Peters, H. (1976). Intrauterine gonadal development. *Fertil. Steril.*, **27**, 493–9
3. Patten, B.M. (1964). The development of the urogenital system. In Patten, B.M. (ed.) *Foundations of Embryology*, pp. 180–512. (New York: McGraw-Hill)
4. Yding Andersen, C., Byskov, A.G. and Grinsted, J. (1983). Growth pattern of the sex ducts in foetal

mouse hermaphrodites. *J. Embryol. Exp. Morphol.*, **73**, 59–68

5. Taguchi, O., Cunha, G.R., Lawrence, W.D. and Robboy, S.J. (1984). Timing and irreversibility of Müllerian duct inhibition in the embryonic reproductive tract of the human male. *Dev. Biol.*, **106**, 394–8

6. Wartenberg, H., Breucker, H., Holstein, A.F., Dvorák, M. and Tesarík, J. (1990). Entwicklung der Genitalorgane und Bildung der Gameten. In Hindrichsen, K.V. (ed.) *Human Embryologie*, pp. 745–822. (Berlin, Heidelberg, New York: Springer-Verlag)

7. Moore, K.L. and Persuad, T.V.N. (1993). The urogenital system. In Moore, K.L. and Persuad, T.V.N. (eds.) *The Developing Human. Clinically Orientated Embryology*, pp. 265–303. (Philadelphia, London, Tokyo: W.B. Saunders)

8. Barberini, F., Makabe, S., Correr, S., Luzi, A. and Motta, P.M. (1994). An ultrastructural study of epithelium differentiation in the human fetal Fallopian tube. *Acta Anat.*, **151**, 207–19

9. Grünnwald, P. (1941). The relation of the growing Müllerian duct to the Wolffian duct and its importance for the genesis of malformations. *Anat. Rec.*, **82**, 1–19

10. Arey, L.B. (1965). The genital system. In Arey, L.B. (ed.) *Developmental Anatomy*, pp. 315–41. (Philadelphia: W.B. Saunders)

11. Wartenberg, H. (1985). Morphological studies on the role of the periductal stroma in the regression of the human male Müllerian duct. *Anat. Embryol. (Berl).*, **171**, 311–23

12. Kobayashi, S. (1984). Induction of Müllerian duct derivatives in testicular feminized (Tfm) mice by prenatal exposure to diethylstilbestrol. *Anat. Embryol.*, **169**, 35–9

13. McLaren, A. (1960). Of MIS and the mouse. *Nature (London)*, **345**, 111

14. Behringer, R.R., Cate, R.L., Froelick, G.J., Palmiter, R.D. and Brinster, R.L. (1990). Abnormal sexual development in transgenic mice chronically expressing Müllerian inhibiting substance. *Nature (London)*, **345**, 167–70

15. George, F.W. and Wilson, J.D. (1978). Conversion of androgen to estrogen by human fetal ovary. *J. Clin. Endocrinol. Metab.*, **47**, 550–5

16. Josso, N. (1934). Fetal sexual differentiation in mammals. *Ped. Ann.*, **3**, 67–79

17. Josso, N. (1977). The antiMüllerian hormone. *Rec. Prog. Horm. Res.*, **33**, 117–67

18. Vigier, B., Watrin, F., Magre, S., Tran, D. and Josso, N. (1987). Purified bovine AMH induces a characteristic freemartin effect in fetal rat prospective ovaries exposed to it *in vitro*. *Development*, **100**, 43–55

19 Acién, P. (1992). Embryological observations on the female genital tract. *Hum. Reprod.*, **7**, 437–45

20. Robboy, S.J., Taguchi, O. and Cunha, G.R. (1982). Normal development of the human female reproductive tract and alterations resulting from experimental exposure to diethylstilbestrol. *Hum. Pathol.*, **13**, 190–8

21. Carlson, B.M. (1981). The development of the urogenital system. In Carlson, B.M. (ed.) *Patten's Foundations of Embryology*, pp. 440–79. (New York: McGraw-Hill)

22. Cunha, G.R., Shannon, J.M., Taguchi, O., Fujii, H. and Meloy, B.A. (1983). Epithelial–mesenchymal interactions in hormone-induced development. In Sawyer, R.H. and Fallon, J.F. (eds.) *Epithelial–Mesenchymal Interactions in Development*, pp. 51–74. (New York: Praeger Publishers)

23. Cunha, G.R., Chung, L.W.K., Shannon, J.M. and Reese, B.A. (1980). Stromale–epithelial interactions in sex differentiation. *Biol. Reprod.*, **22**, 19–42

24. Cunha, G.R. and Fujii, H. (1981). Stromal–parenchymal interactions in normal and abnormal genital tract. In Herbst, A.L. and Bern, H.A. (eds.) *Developmental Effects of Diethylstilbestrol (DES) in Pregnancy*, pp. 179–93. (New York: Thieme-Stratton)

25. Byskov, A.G. and Høyer, P.E. (1988). Embryology of mammalian gonads and ducts. In Knobil, E. and Neill, J.D. (eds.) *The Physiology of Reproduction*, Vol. 1, pp. 265–302. (New York: Raven Press)

26. Stumpf, W.E., Narbaitz, R. and Sar, M. (1980). Estrogen receptors in the fetal mouse. *J. Steroid Biochem.*, **12**, 55–64

27. Agduhr, E. (1927). Studies on the structure and development of the bursa ovarica and the tuba uterina in the mouse. *Acta Zool.*, **8**, 1–133

28. Brenner, R.M. (1971). Ciliogenesis in the primate oviduct. In Sherman, A.I. (ed.) *Pathways to Conception. The Role of the Cervix and the Oviduct in Reproduction*, pp. 50–66. (Springfield: Charles Thomas)

29. Konishi, I., Fijii, S., Parmley, T.H. and Mori, T. (1987). Development of ciliated cells in the human fetal oviduct: an ultrastructural study. *Anat. Rec.*, **219**, 60–8

30. Komatsu, M. and Fujita, H. (1978). Electron-microscopic studies on the development and aging of the oviduct epithelium of mice. *Anat. Embryol.*, **152**, 243–59

31. Patek, E., Nilsson, L. and Joha, E. (1972). Scanning electron microscopic study of the human Fallopian tube. Report II. Fetal life, reproductive life, and postmenopause. *Fertil. Steril.*, **23**, 719–33

32. Pitynski, K., Litwin, J.A., Nowogradzka-Zagorska, M., Gorczyca, J. and Miodonski, A.J. (1994). The vascular architecture of human fetal oviduct: a scanning electron microscopic study of corrosion casts. *Hum. Reprod.*, **9**, 1958–63

33. Hashimoto, M., Shimoyama, T., Kosaka, M., Komori, A., Hirasawa, T., Yokoyama, Y. and Akashi, K. (1962). Electron microscopic studies on the epithelial cells of the human Fallopian tube. Report I. *J. Jpn. Obstet. Gynecol., Soc.*, **9**, 200–9

34. Novak, E. and Everett., H.S. (1928). Cyclical and other variations in the tubal epithelium. *Am. J. Obstet. Gynecol.*, **16**, 499–530

35. Stegner, H.E. (1961). Das Epithel der Tuba Uterina des Neugeborenen: Elektronenmikroskopische Befunde. *Z. Zellforsch.*, **55**, 247–62

36. Stegner, H.E. (1962). Elektronenmikroskopische Untersuchungen über die Sekretionsmorphologie des Menschlichen Tubenepithels. *Arch. Gynaekol.*, **197**, 351–63

37. Andrews, M.C. (1951). Epithelial changes in the puerperal Fallopian tube. *Am. J. Obstet. Gynecol.*, **62**, 28–37

38. Clyman, M.J. (1966). Electron microscopy of the human Fallopian tube. *Fertil. Steril.*, **17**, 281–301

39. Ferenczy, A., Richart, R.M., Agate, F.J., Purkerson, M.L. and Dempsey, E.W. (1972). Scanning electron microscopy of the human Fallopian tube. *Science*, **175**, 783–5

40. Verhage, H.G., Bareither, H.L. Jaffe, R.C. and Akcar, H. (1979). Cyclic changes in ciliation, secretion and cell height of the oviductal epithelium in women. *Am. J. Anat.*, **156**, 505–23

41. Fawcett, D.W. (1986). Epithelium. In Fawcett, D.W. (ed.) *A Textbook of Histology*, pp. 57–72. (Philadelphia, London, Toronto: W.B. Saunders)

42. Patek, E., Nilsson, L. and Johannisson, E. (1972). Scanning electron microscopic study of the human Fallopian tube. Report I. The proliferative and secretory stages. *Fertil. Steril.*, **23**, 459–65

43. Seki, K., Rawson, J., Eddy, C.A., Smith, N.K. and Paverstein, C.J. (1978). Deciliation in the puerperal Fallopian tube. *Fertil. Steril.*, **29**, 75–83

44. Donnez, J., Casanas-Roux, F., Caprasse, J., Ferin, J. and Thomas, K. (1985). Cyclic changes in ciliation, cell height, and mitotic activity in human tubal epithelium during reproductive life. *Fertil. Steril.*, **43**, 554–9

45. Fredrichson, B. and Björkman, N. (1962). Studies on the ultrastructure of the human oviduct epithelium in different functional states. *Z. Zellforsch. Mikrosk. Anat.*, **58**, 387–96

46. Patek, E., Nilsson, L., Johannisson, E., Helemma, M. and Bout, J. (1973). Scanning electron microscopic study on the human Fallopian tube. Report III. The effect of midpregnancy and of various steroids. *Fertil. Steril.*, **24**, 31–43

47. Gaddum-Rosse, P., Rumery, R.E., Blandau, R.J. and Theirsch, J.B. (1975). Studies on the mucosa of postmenopausal oviducts: surface appearance, ciliary activity and the effect of estrogen treatment. *Fertil. Steril.*, **26**, 951–69

48. Fredrichson, B. and Björkman, N. (1973). Morphologic alterations in the human oviduct epithelium induced by contraceptive steroids. *Fertil. Steril.*, **24**, 19–30

49. Oberti, C., Dabancens, A., Garcia-Huidobro. M., Rodriguez-Bravo, R. and Zanartu, J. (1974). Low dosage oral progestogens to control fertility. II. Morphological modifications in the gonad and oviduct. *Obstet. Gynecol.*, **43**, 285–91

50. Punnonen, R. and Lukola, A. (1981). Binding of estrogen and progestin in the human Fallopian tube. *Fertil. Steril.*, **36**, 610–14

51. Gorski, J., Welshons, W.V., Sakai, D., Hansen, J., Walent, J., Kassis, J., Shull, J., Stack, G. and Campen, C. (1986). Evolution of a model of estrogen action. *Rec. Prog. Horm. Res.*, **42**, 297–329

52. Press, M.F., Nousek-Goeble, N.A., Bur, M. and Greene, G.L. (1986). Estrogen receptor localization in the female genital tract. *Am. J. Pathol.*, **123**, 280–92

53. Press, M.F., Udove, A. and Greene, G.L. (1988). Progesterone receptor distribution in the human endometrium. Analysis using monoclonal antibodies to the human progesterone receptor. *Am. J. Pathol.*, **131**, 112–24

54. Land, J.A. and Arends, J.W. (1992). Immunohistochemical analysis of estrogen and progesterone receptors in Fallopian tubes during ectopic pregnancy. *Fertil. Steril.*, **58**, 335–7

55. Amso, N.N., Crow, J. and Shaw, R.W. (1994). Comparative immunohistochemical study of oestrogen and progesterone receptors in the Fallopian tube and uterus at different stages of the menstrual cycle and the menopause. *Hum. Reprod.*, **9**, 1027–38

Pathology of the Fallopian tube 2

D. S. Heller

NORMAL FALLOPIAN TUBE

The Fallopian tube is 7–12 cm in length, and is anatomically divided proximally to distally into the interstitial portion, isthmic, ampullar and infundibular regions (Figures 1 and 2). There are regional differences in the histology of the tube. The mucosa varies in complexity of folding, being extremely complex in the ampulla and infundibulum, and much less so in the isthmus. Part of the tubal wall is composed of two smooth muscular layers, an inner circular and an outer

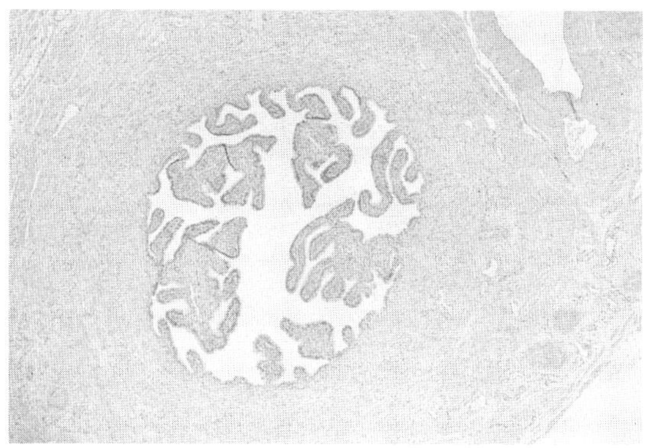

Figure 1 Fallopian tube isthmus – the pattern of mucosal folds is simpler than more distally

longitudinal. The more muscular isthmus contains both an inner and outer longitudinal muscular layer, and a middle circular one. The epithelium of the Fallopian tube is composed of a mixture of three cell types: ciliated, secretory and intercalary cells[1]. The intercalary cells may represent functionally depleted cells, or precursors of the other two cell types.

PROLAPSE OF THE FALLOPIAN TUBE

Occasionally, the Fallopian tube may prolapse into the vaginal vault after vaginal or rarely abdominal hysterectomy[2,3]. On pelvic examination, the tissue looks like the granulation tissue more frequently seen posthysterectomy at the vaginal vault, unless fimbriae are identified. A prolapsed Fallopian tube may cause dyspareunia, and is often accompanied by a bloody or watery discharge. It has been theorized that the cause of tubal prolapse is vaginal vault dehiscence secondary to incomplete healing or trauma[2].

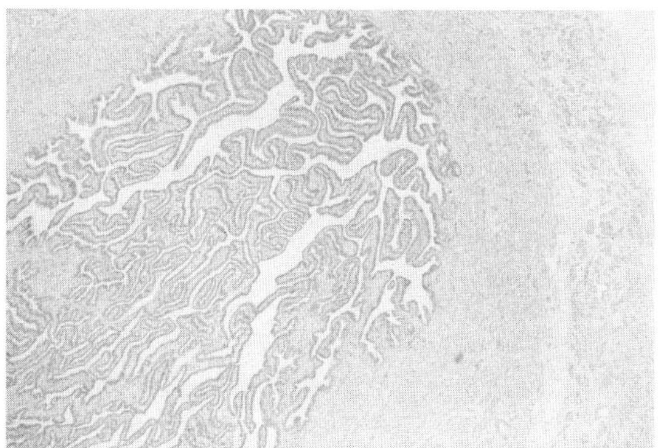
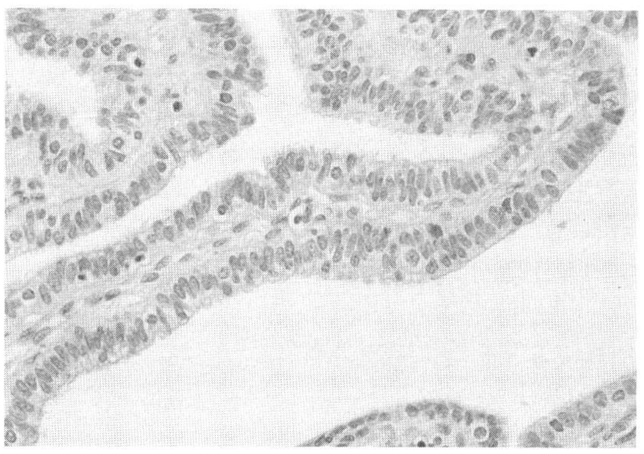

Figure 2 Left, Fallopian tube ampulla – the mucosal folds are complex; right, Fallopian tube epithelium – the epithelium is composed of three cell types: ciliated cells, non-ciliated columnar secretory cells and small intercalary cells

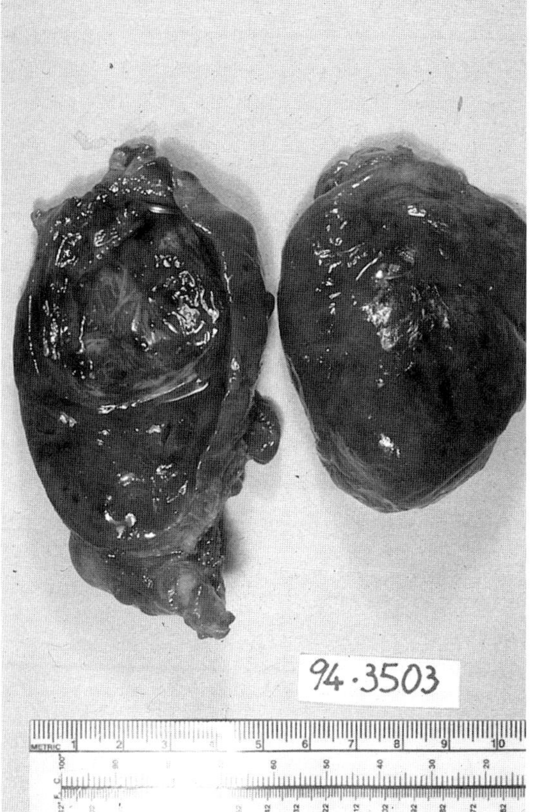

Figure 3 Torsed adnexum

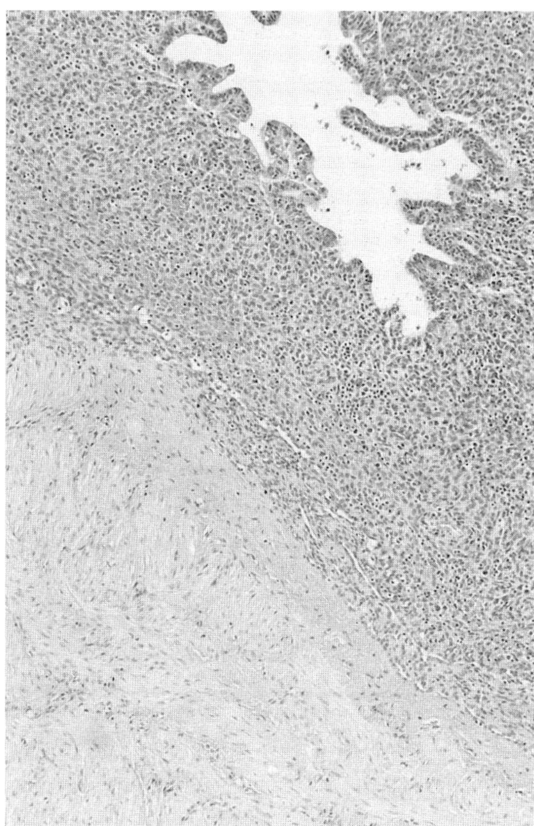

Figure 4 Endometriosis – endometrial glandular epithelium and stroma are present on the serosa of the Fallopian tube

TORSION OF THE FALLOPIAN TUBE

Isolated tubal torsion is uncommon. It appears to involve the fimbriated end, and occurs distal to a compression site, e.g. ligation, ovarian ligament, or adhesion[4]. More commonly, tubal torsion occurs synchronously with ipsilateral ovarian torsion (Figure 3). While the underlying disease process may be obscured by edema, hemorrhage, or necrosis, most torsed adnexa contain an ovarian mass lesion[5]. Out of 35 cases of infarcted uterine adnexa, Demopoulos and colleagues only found five cases with normal ovaries[5]. Of these five cases, two cases of hydrosalpinx were detected. The authors postulated excessive tubal motility secondary to a congenitally abnormally long tube, mesosalpinx, or mesovarium in cases with normal ovaries.

ENDOMETRIOSIS

Endometriosis commonly involves the serosa of the Fallopian tube. Histologically, it is characterized by the presence of both endometrial glandular epithelium and stroma (Figure 4).

INFECTION AND INFLAMMATION OF THE FALLOPIAN TUBE

Acute and chronic salpingitis

Approximately one million American women a year develop pelvic inflammatory disease (PID), with a 25% subsequent infertility rate[6]. Infection is usually ascending, and is commonly associated with *Neisseria gonorrhoeae* or *Chlamydia trachomatis.* Polymicrobial infections are common. Up to 70% of women with infertility secondary to tubal blockage have antibodies to *Chlamydia* in their serum, of which 30–80% never had clinical symp-

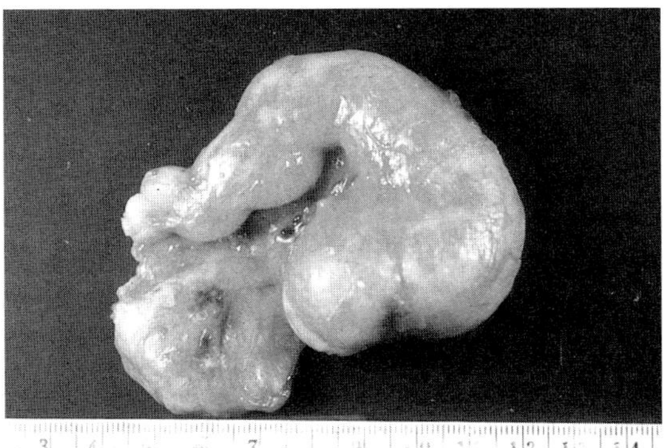

Figure 5 Acute salpingitis – the tube is distended with purulent exudate. The serosal surface is injected

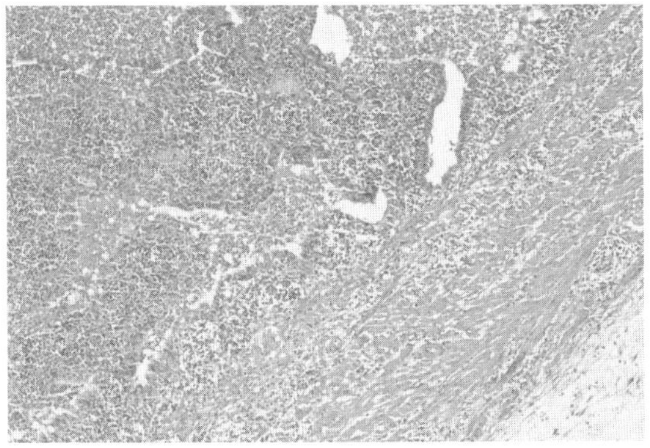

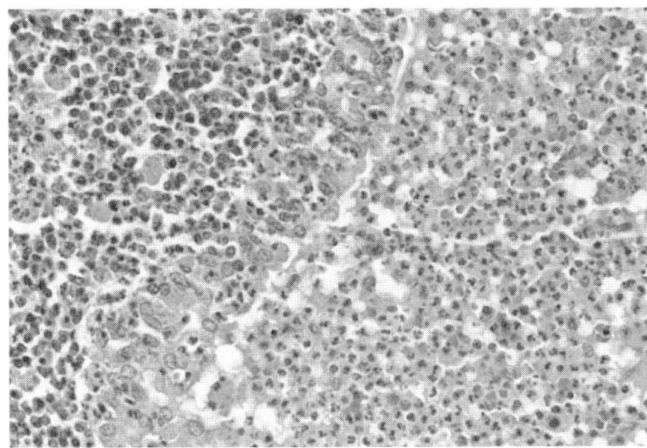

Figure 6 Top and bottom, acute salpingitis – the tubal lumen and subepithelial stroma are infiltrated by polymorphonuclear leukocytes

toms of PID[6]. Women with antibodies to *Chlamydia* have more than a doubled risk of ectopic pregnancy[7]. In a study of patients undergoing microsurgery for distal tubal obstruction, Patton and colleagues found that both patients with silent and a history of clinically overt salpingitis had flattened mucosal folds, loss of epithelial cilia, and secretory cell degeneration[8]. Fifty-two per cent of the overt cases of PID and 57% of the silent PID patients had antibodies to *Chlamydia trachomatis* in this study. Acute salpingitis is characterized grossly by a swollen edematous tube. Vascular congestion may be noted on the serosal surface. The tube may remain patent, or the fimbria may seal, leading to a pyosalpinx (Figure 5). Histologically, an acute inflammatory exudate composed primarily of polymorphonuclear leukocytes is present in the tubal lumen and within the subepithelial stroma (Figure 6). The tubal folds agglutinate. At times, a tubo-ovarian abscess may form, and may require surgical intervention (Figure 7). Chronic salpingitis is characterized by a variable infiltrate of chronic inflammatory cells (Figure 8). The tubal folds often fuse, leading to follicular salpingitis (Figure 9). A fertilized ovum trapped in one of these blind passages is a postulated mechanism of increased ectopic pregnancy risk. After resolution of a pyosalpinx, the accumulation of serous fluid replacing the purulent exudate is termed hydrosalpinx. In hydrosalpinx, the tube may be markedly dilated, with severe loss of the tubal folds (Figures 10 and 11).

Granulomatous salpingitis

The most common cause of granulomatous salpingitis is tuberculosis. Other possible etiologies include actinomyces, some parasites, sarcoidosis, Crohn's disease and foreign body reaction.

Salpingitis secondary to actinomyces

Actinomyces, usually associated with the presence of an intrauterine device (Figure 12), may cause salpingitis, with a propensity for formation of tubo-ovarian abscesses[9].

Tuberculous salpingitis

The incidence of pelvic tuberculosis differs widely in different areas of the world. It has been estimated as being responsible for 19% of female infertility in India, but less than 1% in North America[10]. The genital tract may be involved by hematogenous spread of pulmonary tuberculosis which is probably the most common mode of spread. Lymphatic or direct spread from extrapulmonary tuberculosis may also occur[11]. The

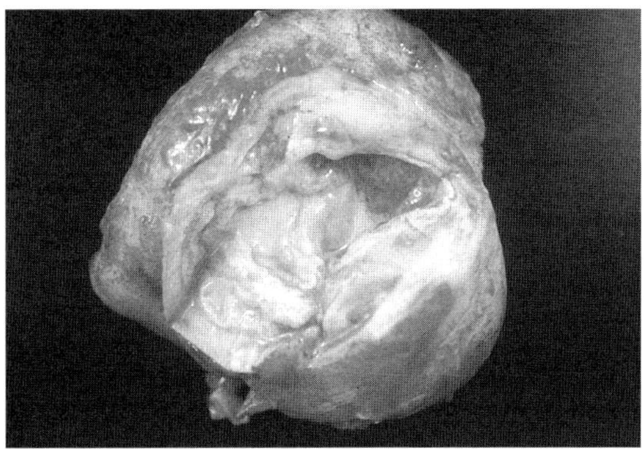

Figure 7 Tubo-ovarian abscess

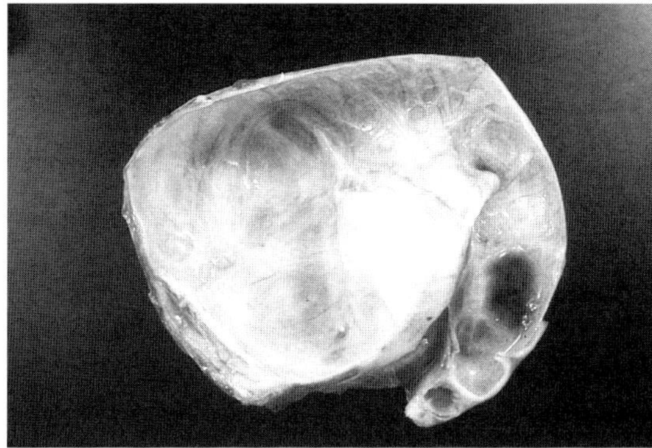

Figure 10 Hydrosalpinx – the tube is markedly dilated

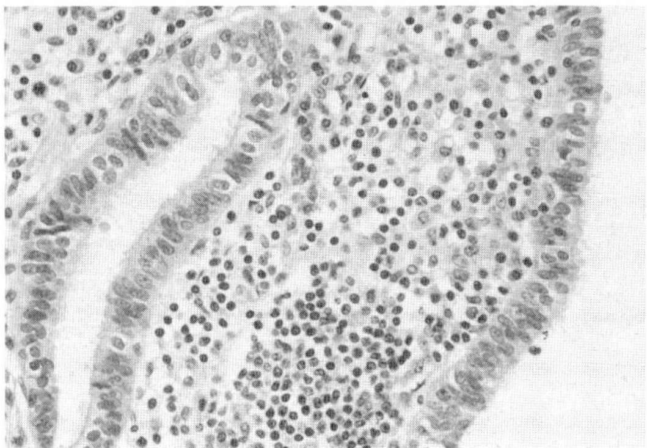

Figure 8 Chronic salpingitis – a chronic inflammatory infiltrate is present

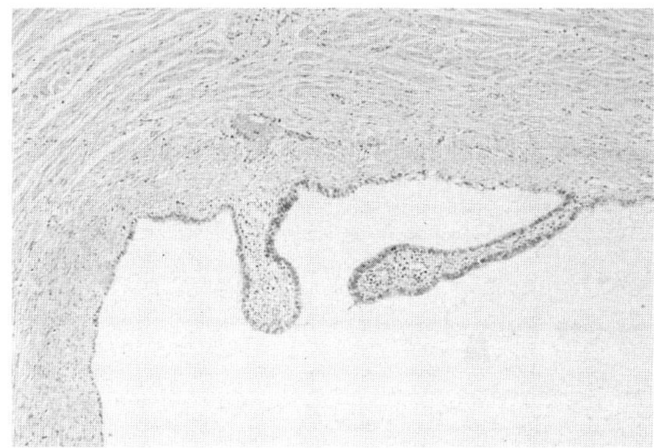

Figure 11 Hydrosalpinx – the tubal epithelium is severely flattened

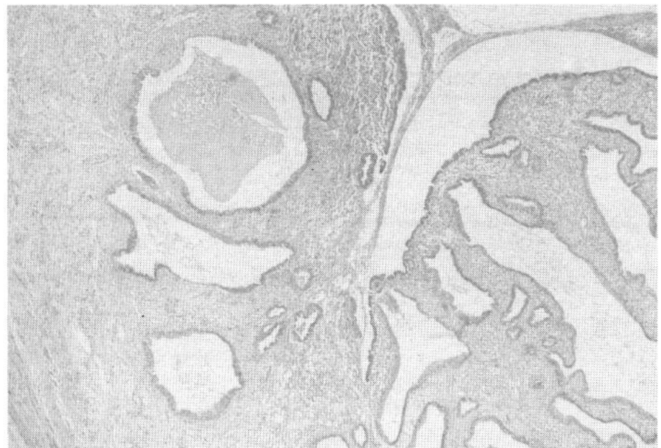

Figure 9 Follicular salpingitis – the tubal folds have fused, forming cystic spaces

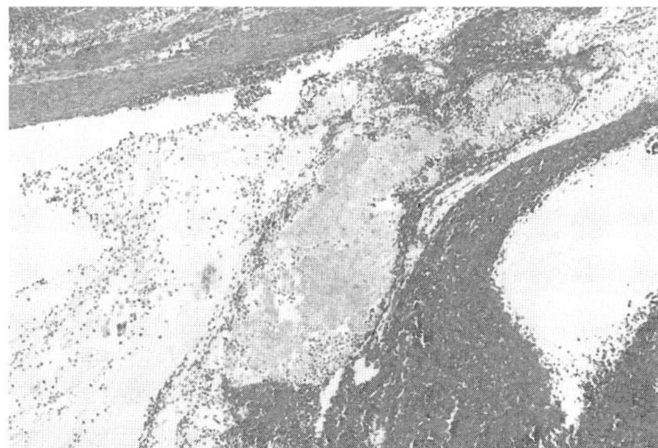

Figure 12 Actinomyces – the typical sulfur granule (Actinomyces colony) is seen on this endocervical curettage specimen

tube is almost always affected, and it may subsequently involve the endometrium and/or ovary. Symptoms are non-specific and include infertility, pain, abnormal uterine bleeding and malaise. Diagnosis may be difficult. Findings on hysterosalpingography are non-specific, and may include midtubal obstruction, multiple tubal constrictions, calcified pelvic lymph nodes, rigid

'pipestem' Fallopian tubes, tubal diverticula and endometrial filling defects[10]. Diagnosis can sometimes be made by endometrial histology or culture; however, not all cases have endometrial involvement. At laparotomy, the tubes may be either swollen but patent, or the pelvis may be studded with tubercles and dense adhesions[10].

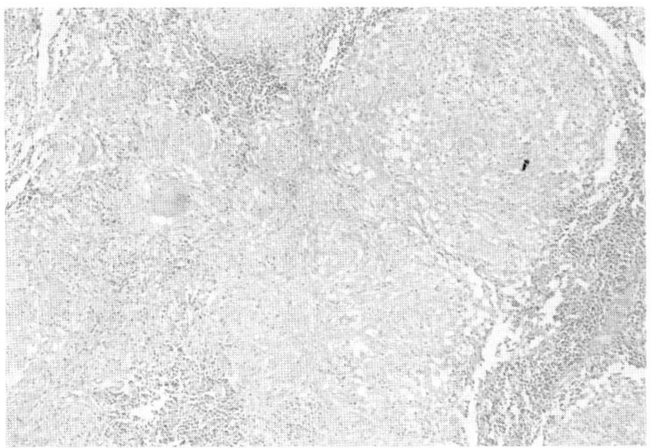

Figure 13 Tuberculosis – caseating granulomas, with central necrosis surrounded by epithelioid cells and Langhans' giant cells

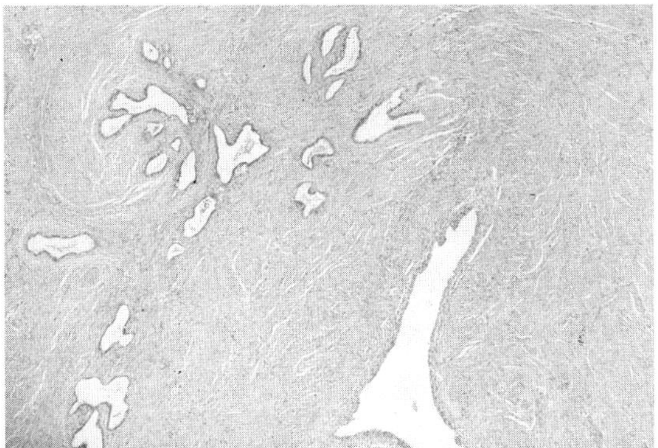

Figure 14 Salpingitis isthmica nodosa – the central tubal lumen is surrounded by epithelial-lined glandular spaces surrounded by hypertrophied smooth muscle. Many of these peripheral glands actually communicate with the central lumen

Histologically, tuberculosis is characterized by caseating granulomas (Figure 13) composed of epithelioid cells and Langhans' giant cells around a necrotic center. A special stain for acid-fast bacilli may reveal organisms if the counts are very high, but is much less sensitive than culture.

SALPINGITIS ISTHMICA NODOSA

Salpingitis isthmica nodosa, initially thought to be inflammatory, is of uncertain etiology. It is associated with infertility and ectopic pregnancy, but a causal relationship has not been established[12]. Theories of origin proposed have included congenital (widely discounted), infection, formation of diverticula similar to the theoretical mechanism of adenomyosis, and tubal spasm[11].

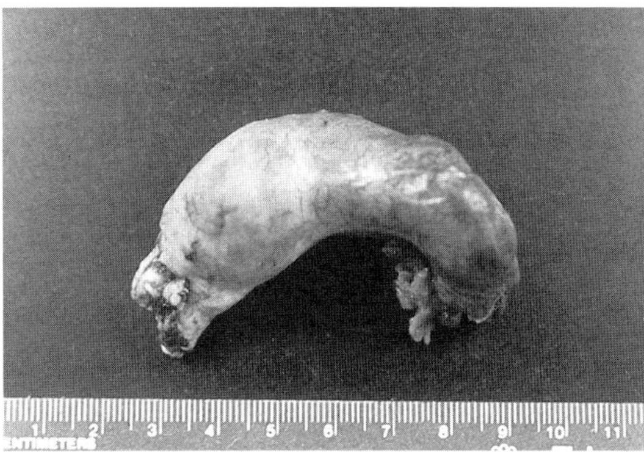

Figure 15 Ectopic pregnancy – in early tubal ectopic pregnancy, a hemorrhagic tubal swelling may be seen

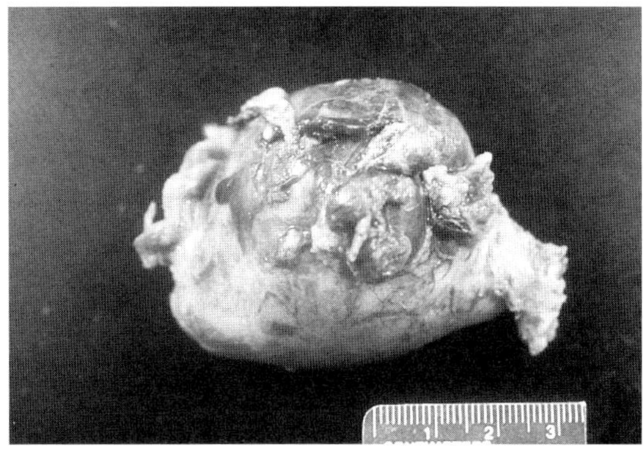

Figure 16 Ectopic pregnancy – as the tubal ectopic progresses, the tube can become markedly distended, and eventually rupture

Grossly, subserosal nodules ranging in size from several millimeters to 2 centimeters may be seen in the isthmic region of the tube[12]. Histologically, on cross-section, multiple lumena are seen surrounding the normal tubal lumen. These are encircled by concentric hypertrophied smooth muscle (Figure 14). Salpingitis isthmica nodosa is essentially analogous to diverticula of the colon or adenomyosis, in that there may be connections to the central tubal lumen[12].

ECTOPIC PREGNANCY

Fallopian tubes examined at the time of resection for ectopic pregnancy show an increased incidence of salpingitis isthmica nodosa and chronic salpingitis[13]. Grossly, the tube may be either mildly enlarged and engorged, or may become markedly dilated (Figures 15 and 16). Most tubal ectopic pregnancies occur in the ampullary region[11]. The

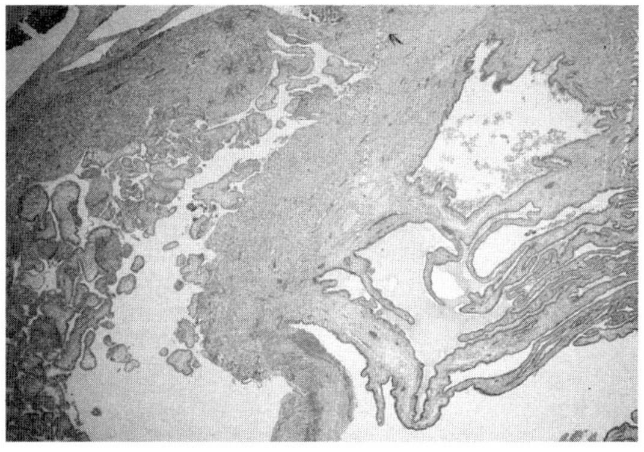

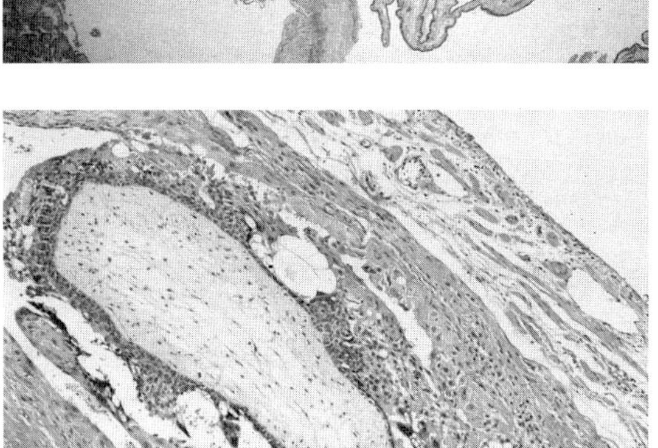

Figure 17 Top and bottom, ectopic pregnancy – immature placental tissue in Fallopian tube

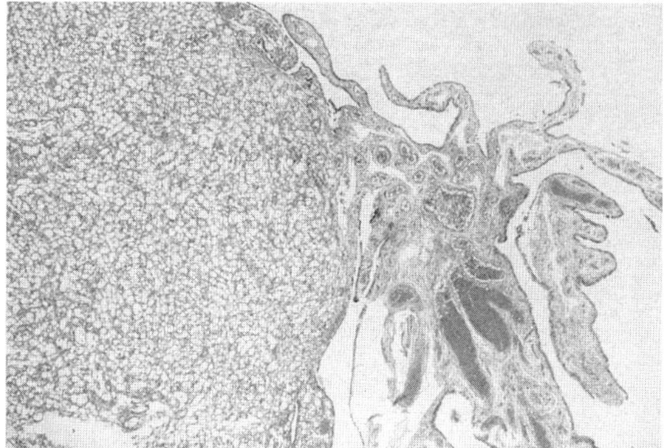

Figure 18 Top, adenomatoid tumor – the tumor is well circumscribed; bottom, adenomatoid tumor – the tumor is composed of slit-like spaces lined by flattened cells of probable mesothelial origin

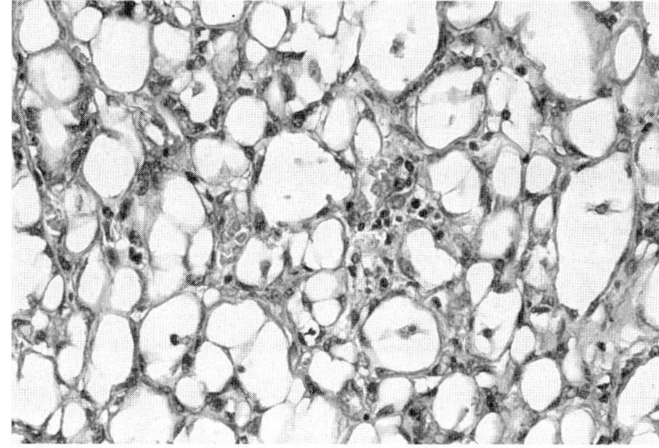

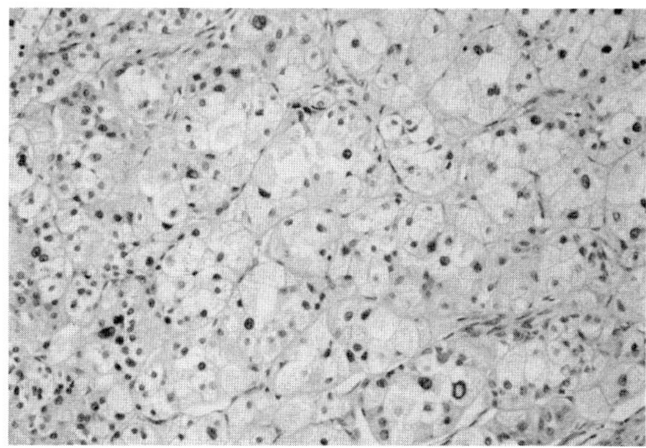

Figure 19 Adrenal cortical rest – a well-circumscribed nodule composed of adrenal cortical cells is sometimes present in the wall of the Fallopian tube. Adrenal medulla is not present

tube may be ruptured or unruptured. Histologically, in an unruptured tubal ectopic, immature placental tissue and occasionally fetal tissue may be seen (Figure 17). If rupture occurs, the products of conception may be extruded into the peritoneal cavity. In these cases, as well as in cases of tubal abortion, it is more difficult to document histologically the ectopic pregnancy. In cases without fetal or placental tissue, the implantation site should be sought. At times, only hematosalpinx may be documented. Only a blood clot may be identifiable in some cases when the tubal contents are examined after linear salpingostomy. In these cases, clinical follow-up of the serum β-human chorionic gonadotropin is indicated.

ADENOMATOID TUMOR

Adenomatoid tumors may arise in the Fallopian tube, in a subserosal location. These benign tumors are usually incidental findings, but may compress the tubal lumen. They are generally small, well-circumscribed single nodules. Histologically, plexiform, tubular and canalicular patterns may be seen (Figure 18). Histochemistry and electron microscopy support a mesothelial origin[14].

18

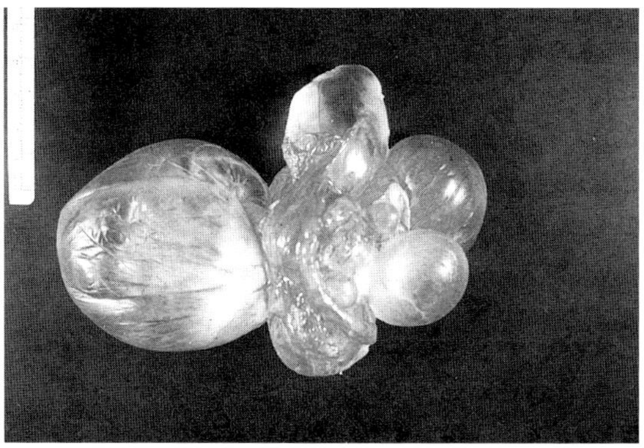

Figure 20 Hydatids of Morgagni – these small paratubal cysts are often incidental findings

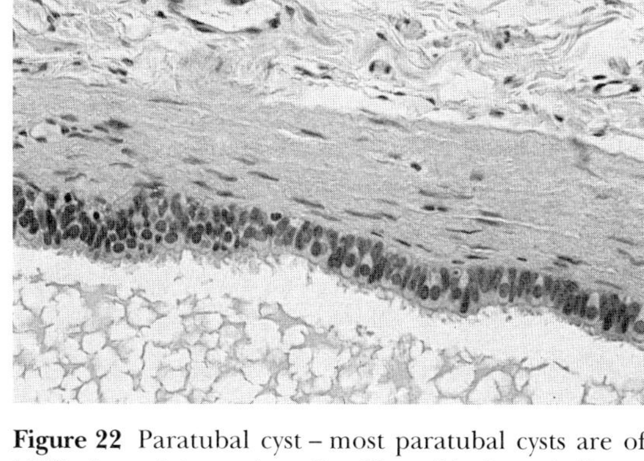

Figure 22 Paratubal cyst – most paratubal cysts are of Müllerian origin, and are lined by epithelium similar to that of the Fallopian tube

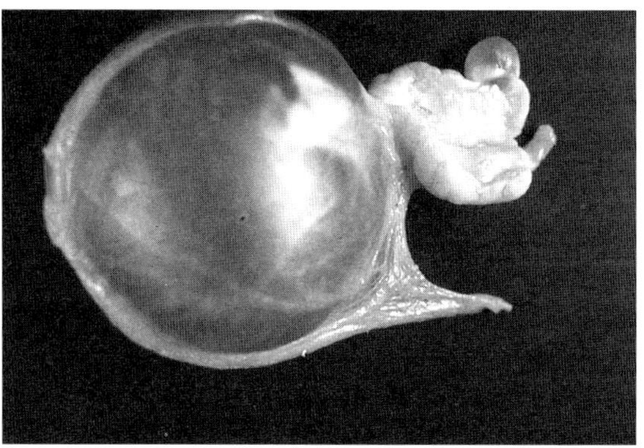

Figure 21 Paratubal cyst – paratubal cysts may occasionally be large enough to present as a pelvic mass

ADRENAL RESTS

Occasionally, adrenal cortical rests may be seen in the Fallopian tube (Figure 19), and are usually incidental findings.

PARATUBAL CYSTS*

Paratubal cysts are of paramesonephric, mesonephric, or mesothelial origin. In a study of 79 paratubal cysts, Samaha and Woodruff[15] found 60 to be of paramesonephric origin, 19 of mesothelial origin, and none of mesonephric origin. Most paratubal cysts are incidental findings, commonly in the third to fourth decade, although if large they may present as a pelvic mass (Figures 20 and 21). It is unclear whether there is an increased incidence among infertile patients[15].

Histologically, paratubal cysts of para-mesonephric origin are lined by an epithelium similar to Fallopian tube epithelium, a non-stratified columnar lining composed of ciliated, secretory and intercalary cells (Figure 22). The cyst wall is usually a thin smooth muscle layer. The epithelium may fall into papillary folds, mimicking the architecture of the Fallopian tube. Paratubal cysts of mesothelial origin are lined by a flat epithelial layer, and are surrounded by fibro-fatty tissue. Paratubal cysts of mesonephric origin have a thicker muscular wall than those of para-mesonephric origin, and are lined by a low cuboidal non-secretory epithelium[15].

Serous neoplasms can occur in the paratubal region. These are usually benign (Figure 23), although low malignant potential and malignant serous tumors have been described.

ADNEXAL TUMOR OF PROBABLE WOLFFIAN ORIGIN

These rare tumors are considered to be of low malignant potential, without established histological predictors of behavior[16]. Histologically, they may be solid epithelioid sheets, or composed of tubules lined by columnar cells.

---

* From Heller, D. and Greenebaum, E. Intraperitoneal Gynecologic Cytology – Aspiration of ovarian and adnexal cysts and peritoneal washings with clinical and pathologic correlations. ASCP National Meeting Workshop 1993.

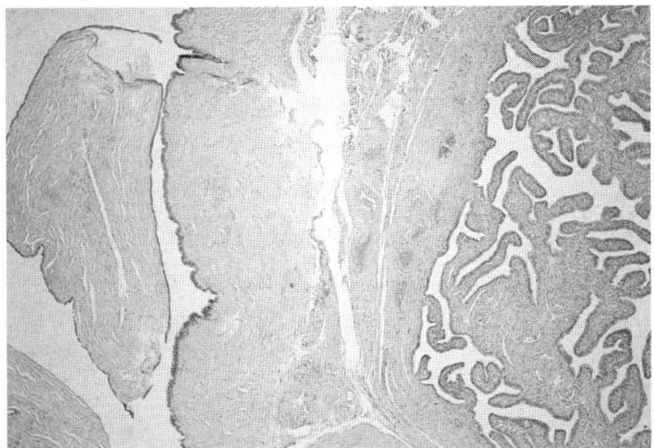

Figure 23 Adenofibroma – occasionally a benign neoplasm such as this adenofibroma or a malignancy can arise in a paratubal cyst

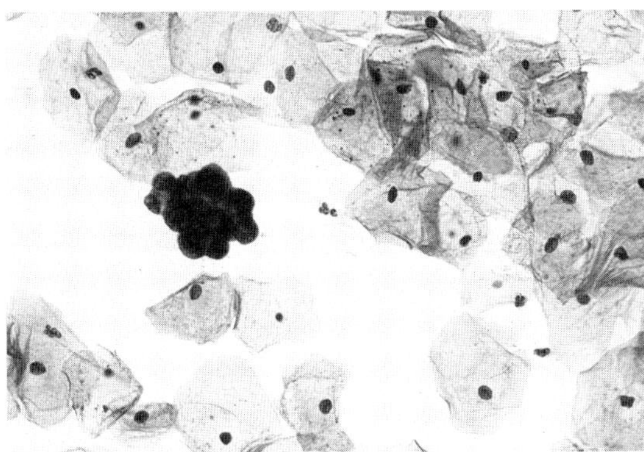

Figure 24 Papanicolaou smear showing atypical glandular clusters suspicious for adenocarcinoma. The patient was found at hysterectomy to have carcinoma *in situ* of the Fallopian tube (see Figure 27)

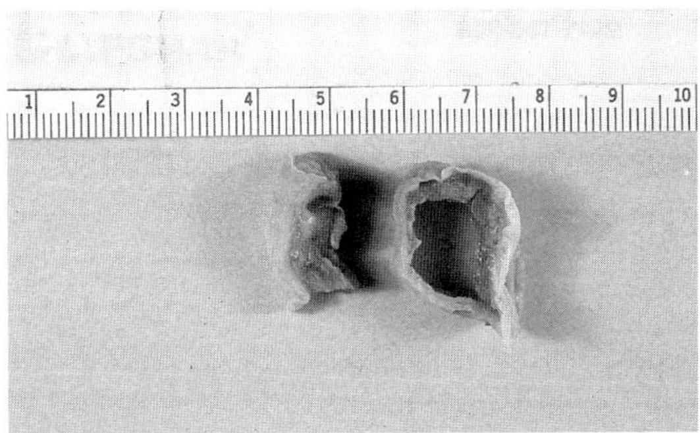

Figure 25 Carcinoma of the Fallopian tube – cross-sections of tube showing intraluminal growth

CARCINOMA OF THE FALLOPIAN TUBE

Fallopian tube carcinoma represents less than 0.5% of gynecological cancer[9]. The mean age of the patients is 56.7 years[17].

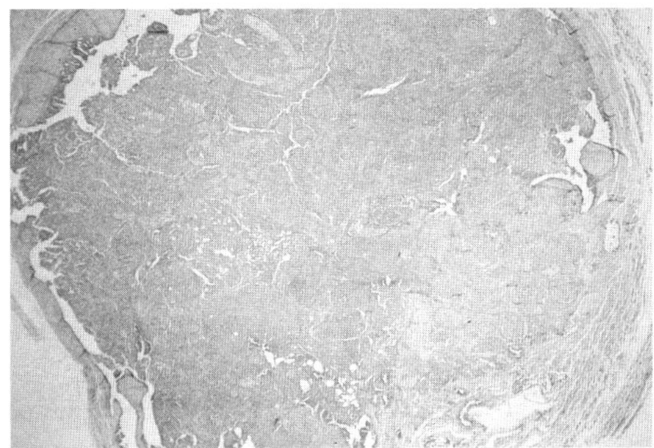

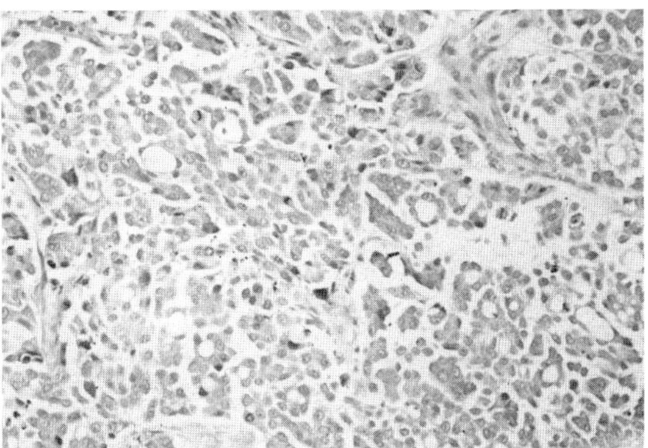

Figure 26 Carcinoma of the Fallopian tube – most tubal carcinomas are either papillary serous (bottom) or poorly differentiated (top) tumors

Clinical presentation is similar to ovarian carcinoma; symptoms are usually non-specific and diagnosis is often late in the disease process. Symptoms and signs may include pain, mass and serosanguinous vaginal discharge ('Latzko's triad'), or vaginal bleeding[17]. Hydrops tubae perfluens, the passage of blood-tinged watery fluid vaginally after an episode of cramping, is uncommon. Rarely, tubal carcinoma may be diagnosed on a Papanicolaou smear (Figure 24). Ca-125 may be elevated[17].

Grossly, the tumor arises from tubal mucosa, and the tube may be dilated, with or without tumor on the external surface (Figure 25).

Bilaterality is present in 10–26%, and while this may represent metastatic spread, it is felt by some to be due to multifocal disease[17]. In the presence of ovarian involvement, it may be difficult to establish the tube as the primary site. Sedlis[18] established the following criteria for a Fallopian tube primary:

(1) The tumor arises from the endosalpinx;

(2) It reproduces the epithelium of the tubal mucosa;

(3) A transition is present between benign and malignant tubal epithelium, and

(4) Endometrial and/or ovarian tumor is absent or less.

Histologically, most Fallopian tube carcinomas are either papillary serous or undifferentiated (Figure 26). As Müllerian epithelium is multipotential, endometrioid, clear cell, adenosquamous, squamous, transitional and glassy cell patterns have also been described[9].

Prognosis overall is poor; early-stage disease has a 5-year survival of only about 50%[19]. Up until recently, FIGO staging for ovarian carcinoma was used, however, in 1991, in an attempt better to evaluate Fallopian tube cancer, a separate staging was proposed[20] (Table 1). This staging takes into consideration the presence of a basement membrane between the tubal epithelium and wall, allowing for a carcinoma *in situ* category (Figure

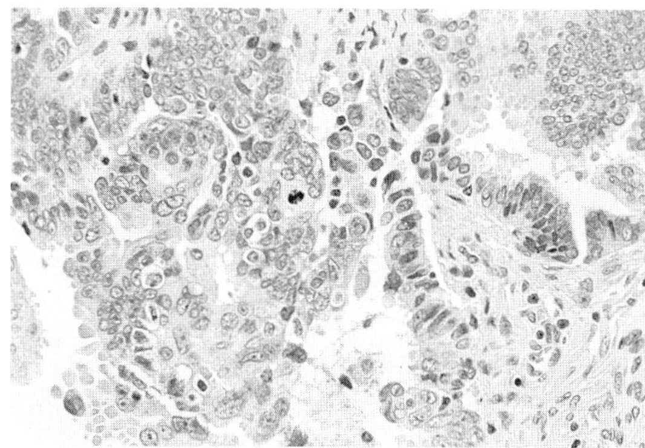

Figure 27 Carcinoma *in situ* of the Fallopian tube – the neoplastic process is confined to the epithelium

27). With this staging, it has been established that prognosis drops rapidly from stage 0 (carcinoma *in situ*) to stage I (50% 5-year survival)[19].

The distinction between carcinoma *in situ* of the Fallopian tube and benign epithelial proliferations rests on mitotic activity. Moore and Enterline[21] have described benign proliferative epithelial lesions showing nuclear crowding, stratification, loss of polarity, atypia, eosinophilic cells and papil-

Table 1   FIGO staging of Fallopian tube carcinoma[20]

0	Carcinoma *in situ* (limited to tubal mucosa)
I	Limited to Fallopian tubes
IA	Growth limited to one tube with extension into submucosa and/or muscularis but not penetrating serosal surface, no ascites
IB	Growth limited to both tubes with extension into submucosa and/or muscularis but not penetrating serosal surface, no ascites
IC	IA or IB with extension to or through serosa or with positive ascites or washings
II	Growth involving one or both Fallopian tubes with pelvic extension
IIA	Extension and or metastasis to uterus and/or ovaries
IIB	Extension to other pelvic tissues
IIC	IIA or IIB with positive ascites or washings
III	Tumor involving one or both Fallopian tubes with peritoneal implants outside pelvis and/or positive retroperitoneal or inguinal nodes. Superficial liver metastasis equals stage III. Tumor appears limited to true pelvis but with histologically proven malignant extension to small bowel or omentum
IIIA	Tumor grossly limited to true pelvis with negative nodes but with histologically confirmed microscopic seeding of abdominal peritoneal surfaces
IIIB	Tumor involving one or both tubes with histologically confirmed implants of abdominal peritoneal surfaces, none exceeding 2 cm in diameter. Lymph nodes negative
IIIC	Abdominal implants > 2 cm in diameter and/or positive retroperitoneal or inguinal nodes
IV	Growth involving one or both Fallopian tubes with distant metastases. If pleural effusion is present, cytologic fluid must be positive for malignant cells. Parenchymal liver metastases

lary projections. Mitotic activity was rare. They noted an association with salpingitis, and felt the lesions did not represent carcinoma *in situ*.

OTHER UNCOMMON TUMORS OF THE FALLOPIAN TUBE

Tumors of the Fallopian tube are classified as epithelial, mixed epithelial–mesenchymal and mesenchymal according to the World Health Organization[11]. Benign epithelial tumors include adenomas and papillomas. As mentioned previously, a variety of malignant epithelial tumors can arise from the multipotential Müllerian epithelium of the Fallopian tube. Mixed epithelial–mesenchymal tumors include adenomyoma, adenofibroma and malignant mixed mesodermal tumors. Mesenchymal lesions include leiomyomas and leiomyosarcomas.

References

1. Eddy, C.A. and Pauerstein, C.S. (1980). Anatomy and physiology of the Fallopian tube. *Clin. Obstet. Gynecol.*, **23**,1177–93
2. Ellsworth, H.S., Harris, J.W., McQuarrie, H.G., Stone, R.A. and Anderson, A.E. (1973). Prolapse of the Fallopian tube following vaginal hysterectomy. *J. Am. Med. Assoc.*, **224**, 891–2
3. Sapan, I.P. and Solberg, N.S. (1973). Prolapse of the Fallopian tube after abdominal hysterectomy. *Obstet. Gynecol.*, **42**, 26–32
4. Bernardus, R.E., Van Der Slikke, J.W., Roex, A.J.M., Dijkhuizen, G.H. and Stolk, J.G. (1984). Torsion of the Fallopian tube: some considerations on its etiology. *Obstet. Gynecol.*, **64**, 675–8
5. Demopoulos, R.I., Bigelow, B. and Vasa, U. (1978). Infarcted uterine adnexa-associated pathology. *NY State J. Med.*, **78**, 2027–9
6. McCormack, W.M. (1994). Pelvic inflammatory disease. *N. Engl. J. Med.*, **330**, 115–19
7. Chow, J.M., Yonekura, M.L., Richwald, G.A., Greenland, S., Sweet, R.L. and Schachter, J. (1990). The association between *Chlamydia trachomatis* and ectopic pregnancy: a matched pair case–control study. *J. Am. Med. Assoc.*, **263**, 3164–7
8. Patton, D.L., Moore, D.E., Spadoni, L.R., Soules, M.R., Halbert, S.M. and Wang, S.P. (1989). A comparison of the Fallopian tube's response to overt and silent salpingitis. *Obstet. Gynecol.*, **73**, 622–30
9. Thor, A.D., Young, R.H. and Clement, P.B. (1991). Pathology of the Fallopian tube, broad ligament, peritoneum, and pelvic soft tissues. *Hum. Pathol.*, **22**, 856–67
10. Bateman, B.G., Nunley, W.C., Kitchin, J.D. and Fechner, R.E. (1980). Genital tuberculosis in reproductive-age women. A report of two cases. *J. Reprod. Med.*, **31**, 287–90
11. Wheeler, J.E. (1994). Diseases of the Fallopian tube. In Kurman, R.J. (ed.) *Blaustein's Pathology of the Female Genital Tract*, 4th edn., p. 529. (New York: Springer-Verlag)
12. Jenkins, C.S., Williams, S.R. and Schmidt, G.E. (1993). Salpingitis isthmica nodosa: a review of the literature, discussion of clinical significance and consideration of patient management. *Fertil. Steril.*, **60**, 599–607
13. Green, L.K. and Kott, M.L. (1989). Histopathologic findings in ectopic tubal pregnancy. *Int. J. Gynecol. Pathol.*, **8**, 255–62
14. Taxy, J.B., Battifora, H. and Oyasu, R. (1974). Adenomatoid tumors: a light microscopic, histochemical, and ultrastructural study. *Cancer*, **34**, 306–16
15. Samaha, M. and Woodruff, J.D. (1985). Paratubal cysts: frequency, histogenesis, and associated clinical features. *Obstet. Gynecol.*, **65**, 691–3
16. Flanagan, A.M., Kane, J.L. and Norman-Taylor, J.Q. (1987). Female adnexal tumor of probable Wolffian origin. Case report. *Br. J. Obstet. Gynaecol.*, **94**, 270–2
17. Nordin, A.J. (1994). Primary carcinoma of the Fallopian tube: a 20-year literature review. *Obstet. Gynecol. Surv.*, **49**, 349–61
18. Sedlis, A. (1978). Carcinoma of the Fallopian tube. *Surg. Clin. N. Am.*, **58**, 121
19. Klein, M., Rosen, A., Graf, A., Lahousen, M., Kucera, H., Pakisch, B., Vavra, N. and Beck, A. (1994). Primary Fallopian tube carcinoma – a retrospective survey of 51 cases. *Arch. Gynecol. Obstet.*, **255**, 141–6
20. Creaseman, W.T. (1992). Revision in classification by International Federation of Gynecology and Obstetrics. *Am. J. Obstet. Gynecol.*, **167**, 857–8
21. Moore, S.W. and Enterline, H.T. (1975). Significance of proliferative epithelial lesions of the uterine tube. *Obstet. Gynecol.*, **45**, 385–90

The normal Fallopian tube 3

A. Monteagudo, J. P. Lerner and I. E. Timor-Tritsch

INTRODUCTION

The Fallopian tubes, or oviducts, or uterine tubes, are derived from the Müllerian ducts and arise from the cornual end of the uterus. They are a paired organ and their task is to serve as a 'conveyor belt' for the transfer of the oocytes and the sperm for their meeting for conception.

The Fallopian tubes are about 7–12 cm long and are covered by peritoneum which duplicates to form one of its loose attachments, the meso-salpinx, to the broad ligament. Their proximal narrow portion, called the isthmus, has a narrow lumen and a thick muscular wall. Next is the ampullar part which has an expanding lumen and a convoluted endosalpingeal mucosa. The end portion, the infundibulum, is the trumpet-shaped part of the tube ending in the fimbriae which are found close to the ovary. The outer layer of the tube's muscle is composed of longitudinal fibers; the inner layer has fibers oriented in a circular fashion.

The arterial blood supply to the oviducts is derived from the terminal branches of the uterine and the ovarian arteries. The branches of the uterine arteries supply the medial two-thirds of each tube. The ovarian arteries supply the lateral one-third of the tube. The venous drainage parallels the arterial supply. The lymphatic system stands alone, separate from that of the uterus. Drainage occurs through the internal iliac nodes and the aortic nodes surrounding the aorta and the inferior vena cava.

The only sonographically significant anomaly of the Fallopian tubes is that involving the area of the uterine cornua/isthmic portion of the oviduct. Agenesis or rudimentary development of this area leaves the ampulla and the infundibulum unconnected to the uterus. This can lead to a pregnancy in the blind pouch of the affected tube. The exact sonographic diagnosis of this kind of ectopic pregnancy is virtually impossible to make.

The ultrasonic scanning and evaluation of the Fallopian tubes present a true challenge to even the best sonologists/sonographers. One has clearly to distinguish between the sonographic appearance of a normal and that of an abnormal Fallopian tube. The normal Fallopian tube can be imaged only if fluid surrounds it and creates a sonic interface to outline its boundaries[1]. The most proximal part of it can also be imaged in the normal state, since it is held steady by the uterus, which in this case serves as a landmark for finding the cornual, the isthmic and the proximal 1 or 2 cm of the thin proximal part of the tube. If no fluid is present in the pelvis and the tube is normal, the present transvaginal ultrasound technology is not good enough to image its delicate anatomy[2–4]. Additional reasons for the difficulty in finding a normal tube by sonography in the pelvis are in great part due to limitations of physics: the relatively low resolution of the transabdominal transducers and also the anatomic properties of the Fallopian tubes with their changing shape and location within the pelvis.

If the scope of a pelvic scan is to see tubal pathology, the best way to achieve this is by using a transvaginal ultrasound probe with frequencies of 5 MHz or higher.

As mentioned above, the Fallopian tube is an extremely poor sonic reflector. In spite of the fact that we do not expect to see a normal Fallopian tube during a pelvic transvaginal scan, it is important to describe the anatomic area in which, if the tube is affected by pathology, it is anticipated to be seen. This general area extends bilaterally between the lateral wall of the pelvis, the lateral wall of the uterus and close to the ovaries, wherever they can be found. Fanning up and down (anteriorly and posteriorly) alongside the left and right lateral borders of the uterus in the transverse plane ensures that the scan passes through the expected anatomic location of the Fallopian tube[1, 5–7]. This is also the way to detect pathology and, if such pathology is expected, the above-mentioned technique will be useful.

THE NORMAL TUBE: SONOGRAPHIC ASPECTS

In certain instances, some fluid is present in the pelvis. This, usually sonolucent, fluid acts as a contrast medium to highlight the normal Fallopian tube.

(1) At times a certain amount of pelvic fluid is present and this may be enough to highlight portions of the Fallopian tube.

(2) At midcycle, after the release of follicular fluid, at the time of ovulation or immediately after it, parts of the tube may be detectable.

(3) Blood may be present in the pelvis for various reasons such as rupture of the corpus luteum and rupture of an ectopic pregnancy. Such larger amounts of fluid in the pelvis may increase the chance to detect one or both normal Fallopian tubes.

(4) Ascites present in the pelvis, arising from ovarian hyperstimulation or other conditions, may serve as an excellent contrast medium around the Fallopian tube and the fimbriae in order to highlight them.

(5) Fluid originating from infectious processes may also enable us to outline the Fallopian tubes.

If there is fluid in the pelvis, placing the patient into an anti-Trendelenburg position may increase the pooling of even small amounts of fluid and therefore create the acoustic interface for imaging the tube[2, 6].

The most proximal part of the tube just leaving the cornual area of the uterus is characterized as a more or less sonolucent elongated structure clearly connected with the cornual area of the uterus. Its total length may be about 1–2 cm; this is the extent to which this structure can be followed. During the secretory phase of the cycle, the endometrium becomes echogenic. This is the

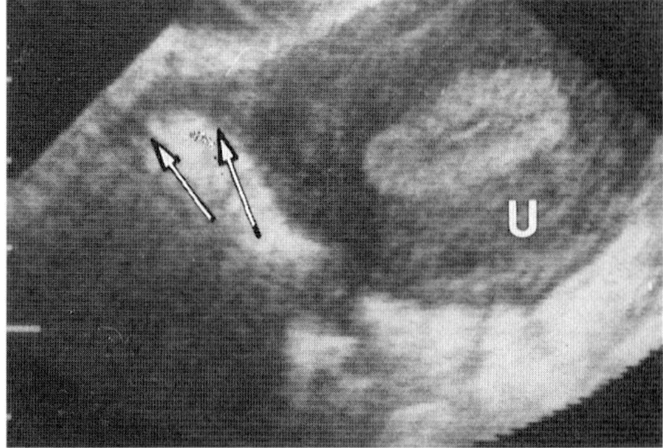

Figure 1 The proximal 1–2 cm of the Fallopian tube (small arrows) can be followed emerging from the uterus (U) by transvaginal sonography

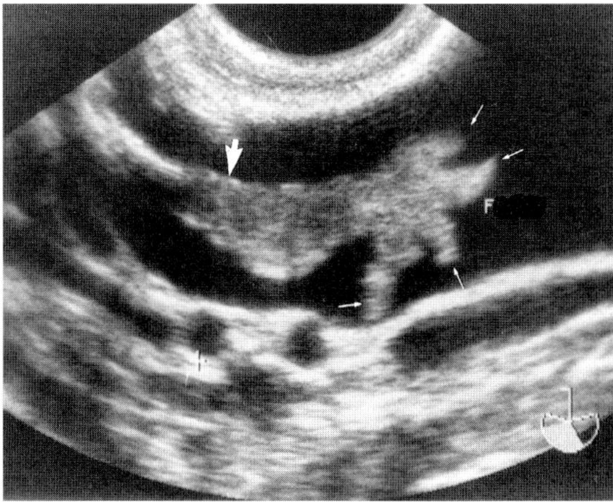

Figure 2 The right Fallopian tube (large arrow) is shown. The small arrows point to the fimbriae (F). Note that a small amount of pelvic fluid is able to highlight the tube

time when this 'shining' echogenic endometrium can be followed through the cornual or isthmic portion into the proximal 1–2 cm of the tube (Figure 1). Its width at this location is about 1 cm at most. If the ampullar part of the tube is seen within the contrasting pelvic fluid described before, it is usually seen as a fusiform, elongated structure which appears to be extremely mobile and changes its place. Towards the ampulla, or further distal, towards the fimbrial end, the width or thickness of the Fallopian tube increases slightly. The free end of the tube demonstrates the typical delicate thin finger-like structures of the fimbria (Figure 2). The fimbriae themselves are usually 1–2 mm in width. By moving the vaginal probe slightly, one can clearly see the undulating

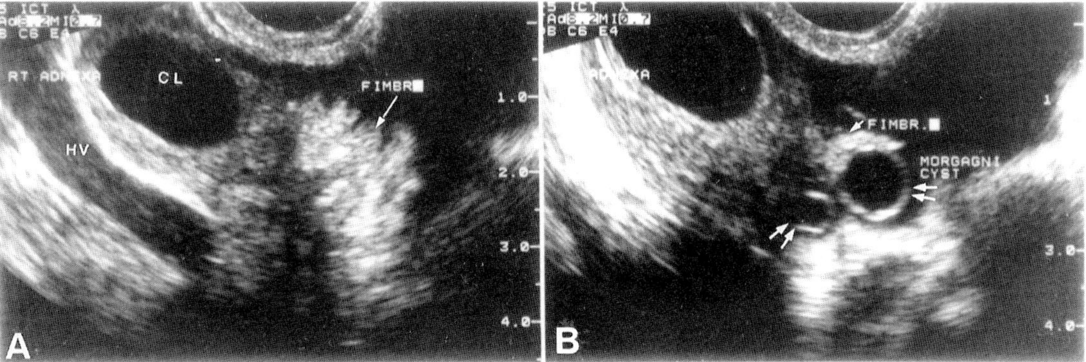

Figure 3 Two successive views of the right adnexa highlighted by cul-de-sac fluid. A, The corpus luteum (CL) is seen in the right ovary above the hypogastric vein (HV). The fimbria floats freely in the fluid. B, Attached to the fimbria two small Morgagni cysts are shown (small double arrows)

movements of these digit-like structures within the fluid.

At times close to the fimbrial end, small 1–1.5 cm thin-walled cysts are seen which contain sonolucent fluid and laparoscopy usually confirms the diagnosis of Morgagni cysts (Figure 3).

For those who would like to see and study the normal Fallopian tube, they should take the opportunity when ascites is diagnosed in a patient scanned for a clinical indication and search the pelvis for the tube. A careful and extremely patient search for the tube floating in the fluid should be done and this may serve as a good opportunity to observe the sonographic appearance of a normal tube. One should, however, remember that, within its normal location among the small bowel and the uterus as well as the ligaments and without the contrasting fluid, the sonographic picture will be entirely different.

Recently, attempts to image the lumen of the Fallopian tubes have been made by injecting contrast material through the cervix and following the hyperechoic sonographic contrast material through the different segments of the oviduct (see Chapter 9). A different way to observe normal patency of the tube is by placing a Doppler window (sample volume) on the expected anatomic location of the oviduct and record the typical flow pattern on the screen.

SUMMARY AND CONCLUSIONS

The normal anatomy of the Fallopian tube is rarely seen by ultrasonography. The best way to attempt to image the tube and its suspected pathology is currently to use high-frequency transvaginal ultrasound techniques. The clinical importance of scanning for tubal patency is yet to be proven on an ongoing basis.

References

1. Timor-Tritsch, I.E. and Rottem, S. (1987). Transvaginal ultrasonographic study of the Fallopian tube. *Obstet. Gynecol.*, **70**, 424–8
2. Timor-Tritsch, I.E., Bar-Yam, Y, Elgali, S. and Rottem, S. (1988). The technique of transvaginal sonography with use of a 6.5 MHz probe. *Am. J. Obstet. Gynecol.*, **158**, 1019
3. Thaler, I., Bruck, A. and Bar-Yam, Y. (1988). The vaginal probe – physical considerations. In Timor-Tritsch, I.E. and Rottem, S. (eds.) *Transvaginal Sonography.* (New York: Elsevier)
4. Thaler, I. and Manor, D. (1990). Transvaginal imaging: applied physical principles and terms. *J. Clin. Ultrasound*, **18**, 235

5. Rottem, S., Thaler, I., Goldstein, I., Timor-Tritsch, I.E. and Brandes, J.M. (1990). Transvaginal sonographic technique: targeted organ scanning without resorting to 'planes'. *J. Clin. Ultrasound*, **18**, 243

6. Timor-Tritsch, I.E., Rottem, S. and Lewit, N.(1991). The Fallopian tubes. In Timor-Tritsch, I.E. and Rottem, S. (eds.) *Transvaginal Sonography*, 2nd edn., pp. 131–44. (New York: Chapman & Hall)

7. Timor-Tritsch, I.E., Rottem, S. and Elgali, S. (1988). How transvaginal sonography is done. In Timor-Tritsch, I.E. and Rottem, S. (eds.) *Transvaginal Sonography*. (New York: Elsevier)

Ultrasonographic aspects of ectopic pregnancy

I. E. Timor-Tritsch, A. Monteagudo and J. P. Lerner

INTRODUCTION

The definition of ectopic pregnancy is a gestation which implants outside the boundaries of the uterine cavity. In the past 20 years, the rate of ectopic pregnancies has increased significantly in the world, and also in the United States. The Center for Disease Control in the United States keeps an accurate track of statistical data regarding ectopic pregnancies. Between the years 1970 and 1987, there was an almost fourfold increase in the incidence of ectopic pregnancy from 4.5 to 16.8 per 1000 pregnancies[1].

In contrast, the fatality rate decreased steeply from 35.5 deaths per 10 000 ectopic pregnancies in 1970 to 3.4 in 1987[1]. In spite of this dramatic decrease in mortality, ectopic pregnancy is still among the leading causes of maternal morbidity and mortality in the United States. Ectopic pregnancy is also responsible for reduced childbearing potential. It is believed that even the existing low maternal death rate can further be reduced if a timely diagnosis and treatment were available[2].

The traditional approach to tubal pregnancy has been the removal of the tube hosting the ectopic pregnancy. However, modern diagnostic tools detect and classify an ectopic pregnancy earlier, and in a more accurate fashion, than in previous years. These advances have brought about a changing trend towards the management process of this disease. The increasing trend towards conservative management of tubal and other pregnancies reflects the attempt to reduce morbidity and preserve fertility. To study the trends in the United States, as far as management of tubal pregnancy is concerned, Young and colleagues[3] scrutinized the American National Hospital Discharge Survey. They revealed that tubal pregnancies managed conservatively, through operative procedures that attempt to preserve the function of the tube, increased from 2% in 1970–1978, to 12% in 1984–1987. The use of diagnostic laparoscopy increased from 10% in 1970–1978, to 33% in 1979–1987, whereas the use of diagnostic laparotomy decreased from 24% to 2%. One should realize that these statistical data were generated before the wide introduction of transvaginal sonography for the early detection of ectopic pregnancies. To our knowledge, there is no updated data source to show an additional improvement in the diagnosis and decrease in the maternal morbidity and mortality rate to reflect the impact of this new diagnostic tool.

As far as the location of ectopic pregnancies is concerned, more than 90% of ectopic pregnancies involve the Fallopian tube; the remaining ectopic gestations implant in the cornual or isthmic area of the tube, in the ovary, the cervix and different sites of the abdominal cavity.

ETIOLOGY

Very little is known about the exact cause of ectopic pregnancies. Several etiologies have been mentioned in the literature; however, few proofs for them exist[4–6]. Some of the functional factors which are throught to interfere with passage of the fertilized egg into the uterine cavity are: the menstrual reflux, the possible external migration of the ovum to a contralateral Fallopian tube, and a disturbed or somewhat altered motility of the Fallopian tube. Among the mechanical factors that have been implicated in the prevention of the movement of the fertilized egg, are the following: low-grade infection of the pelvic contents, which is believed to be the main cause for the faulty implantation of the fertilized egg and/or the embryo, peritubal adhesions as a result of previous pelvic inflammatory disease, and, of course, salpingitis with the partial or total destruction of the tubal mucosa.

LABORATORY PREGNANCY TESTS

The largest addition to the detection and the correct diagnosis of ectopic pregnancies is undoubtedly the introduction of qualitative and quantitative human chorionic gonadotropin (hCG) tests, which are currently available, constantly improved and, hopefully, becoming less and less expensive.

The hCG is first detectable about 9–11 days after conception. However, most blood pregnancy tests which are based on its quantitative assessment are considered to be positive past the level of 10–15 mIu/ml. Right at the outset, we have to define the kind of laboratory test we are using and the units in which the qualitative values are reported. Quantitative biochemical laboratory tests are usually performed by aspirating the patient's blood. There are various standards for reporting hCG levels; one of the most used is the International Reference Preparation (IRP), and another is the Second International Standard (second IS). The difference between the two is that the second IS values are approximately half the IRP values. Lately, several other biochemical laboratory tests have been used and geared towards other subunits or biochemical combinations of the hCG concerned. The second form of hCG determination uses the patient's urine, usually employing monoclonal antibody testing to ascertain the presence of the hCG molecule in the urine. The sensitivity of these tests is quite good and they can detect levels as low as 50 mIu/ml (IRP).

It is not enough to report that a positive test for β-hCG was found. The titer has to be correlated with the sonographic picture. The term 'discriminatory β-hCG level' was coined to express the titer of this pregnancy hormone when a chorionic (gestational) sac was seen in the cavity of a normal (non-fibromatous) uterus. Transabdominal and transvaginal probes have different discriminatory β-hCG levels. For historical reasons, it should be mentioned that, using a transabdominal probe of 3.5 MHz, a normal intrauterine pregnancy is detectable at a level of 6500 mIU/ml (IRP) [7]. Transvaginal probes using 5–7.5 MHz perform much better. They detect the gestation at levels of 1000 (± 200) mIU/ml (IRP) [8–12]. Even though it was suggested that it is possible to discriminate the presence of an ectopic gestation by an abnormal doubling time or a 'flat slope' of the rise in the β-hCG, one should not use this as a reliable diagnostic method. If the ectopic pregnancy is developing and is 'live', it is expected that a careful transvaginal scanning will detect the ectopic sac at discriminatory titers similar to those used in the case of a normal intrauterine pregnancy.

Practically, the discriminatory zone tells us the particular blood level of β-hCG above which a normal intrauterine pregnancy is detected by the current level and technology of ultrasound employed if that pregnancy is implanted in a normal uterus of a woman with a normal body habitus [13]. If the meaning of the previous definition is analyzed, it becomes clear that several factors will affect the level of the β-hCG at which a normal intrauterine pregnancy is detected in the setting the clinician is employing. It is clear that, if a higher resolution ultrasound probe is employed, with the capability of using it transvaginally, the level of β-hCG at which a smaller intrauterine pregnancy will be detected will be much lower, i.e. earlier in the gestation. As opposed to this, even if we employ high-frequency transvaginal ultrasound, a perfectly normal gestational sac implanted in a uterus full of fibroids will not be detected until it grows to a certain level, i.e. the β-hCG will necessarily be higher. The discriminatory β-hCG zone also depends upon the visual acuity, the experience of the observer, the quality of the ultrasound machine and lastly, it will also vary with the different laboratories which perform the tests. It should come as no surprise that, when a different β-hCG test is employed, the discriminatory β-hCG zone will change accordingly.

Discriminatory levels of β-hCG for the appearance of the yolk sac and the fetal heart beats in intrauterine pregnancies have also been suggested (7200 mIU/ml and 11 000 mIU/ml, respectively).

Most normal pregnancies follow a well-known and rising pattern; therefore, if a doubling of the hCG level does not occur every 3 days, the pregnancy can be considered a potential extrauterine gestation. This may warn the clinician of the presence of an abnormal intrauterine gestation, or this may also be an ectopic pregnancy.

One of the explicit advantages of the modern pregnancy tests based on monoclonal antibody testing which are, as said before, extremely sensitive to low hCG levels is that they can be employed in the emergency room or in the office of the gynecologist. This definitely presents an advantage since, by applying this pregnancy test followed up by an office ultrasound examination of the pelvis, a fast and almost always reliable diagnosis of the presence or absence of an abnormal or normal intrauterine pregnancy can be made. In the case of an ectopic pregnancy, the chances of making the diagnosis during the first visit to the gynecologist's office or the emergency room are high.

Before starting to use the clinical value of the discriminatory zone of the β-hCG, one should be familiar with the ultrasound equipment and its level of performance as well as the meaning of the biochemical laboratory test that is used.

It is worth mentioning that another marker of the corpus luteum viability, namely the serum progesterone levels, is at times informative. The progesterone level reflects the function of normal corpus luteum during a normal and viable pregnancy. A level of 25 ng/ml or more is associated with a normal intrauterine gestation in about 97% of the cases[14]. If the level of the progesterone is 5 ng/ml or less, that would indicate that abnormal pregnancy or an early pregnancy failure is present, regardless of its location inside or outside the uterine cavity. It is also suggested that this test would be of help in patients who are uncertain of the date of their menstrual period.

CLINICAL ASPECTS OF ECTOPIC PREGNANCY

It is not in the scope of this text to repeat the clinical features of ectopic pregnancy. These can be found elsewhere. Regardless of the obvious importance of establishing the diagnosis of ectopic pregnancy swiftly and accurately, we have to distinguish between the viewpoint of the imaging specialist and that of the practicing obstetrician/gynecologist. The imaging specialist, because of the nature of his work, is more concerned with the different ultrasonographic appearances of the ectopic pregnancy. Furthermore, the imaging specialist is more conservative in making his/her report as far as the diagnosis is concerned, since, from his vantage point, much of the general clinical picture is missing. He/she has to rely on the scant information gathered while the patient is under ultrasonographic examination and on the even less informative requisition form accompanying the patient. In contrast, recently ultrasound machines have appeared in increasing numbers in the offices and emergency rooms of obstetricians and gynecologists. This enables a different approach to the patient and to their diagnosis by these practitioners. Obviously, in the offices of obstetricians/gynecologists, every patient in her reproductive years complaining of lower abdominal pain, with some degree of vaginal bleeding, will immediately trigger the 'rule-out ectopic' diagnostic algorithm which, of course, includes a sonogram. Regardless of how atypical the complaints of a patient are, the good clinician gathers an initial and careful history about the menstrual periods, previous possible ectopic pregnancies, contraceptive practices, history of pelvic inflammatory diseases, and, above all, of the patient's participation in infertility treatment or assisted reproductive technologies. If there is enough evidence to pursue the diagnostic algorithm of a possible ectopic gestation, the next step will include the performance of a simple pregnancy test which is sensitive and reliable in order to support or to rule out the presence of a pregnancy in the patient. If this pregnancy test is positive, the next obvious step is transvaginal sonography. We have already touched upon β-hCG testing and the possibility of performing serum progesterone measurements.

The next possible diagnostic (and in part therapeutic) procedures are the curettage, laparoscopy and the much debated culdocentesis. The above-mentioned procedures are obviously invasive procedures by which to arrive at the diagnosis.

Curettage

If the patient has a positive hCG test and transvaginal sonography does not show an intrauterine gestation, the approximate age of the pregnancy has to be determined. If the uterus is only slightly enlarged and the level of hCG fails to show an appropriate rise, e.g. a minimum of 66% every 48 h, and the cul-de-sac does not contain a threatening amount of hemorrhage, then curettage and examination of the tissue for chorionic villi is the next step.

This can be done in one of two ways: first, by direct examination of the tissue which is washed under a stream of water (remember that those expert in chorionic villus sampling can detect the presence of 15–20 mg of placental tissue just by examining it with the naked eye in the Petri dish); and second, by sending the specimen for histological examination. The presence of chorionic villi proves an early pregnancy failure and no further testing is necessary. If there is only decidua present, which of course is of maternal origin, the presence of an extrauterine gestation is possible. If no cul-de-sac fluid is seen by transvaginal sonography, a follow-up serum β-hCG should be obtained within 2 days. If the level is declining, an abortion may be the case. This can be complete abortion of an intrauterine pregnancy but could also be an aborting tubal gestation. If the β-hCG is increasing, and assuming that the uterus is empty, then an extrauterine pregnancy is definitely the case. The levels and the trend of the β-hCG will, in these cases, determine the future treatment for the patient.

Laparoscopy

Laparoscopy has always been regarded as the ultimate diagnostic test for ectopic pregnancy. The performance of a meaningful laparoscopic examination requires an experienced operator, sophisticated equipment and an operating room with high-level personnel. All these may not be present at night. The procedure is usually done under general anesthesia. The advantage of laparoscopy is that it can not only diagnose the ectopic pregnancy, but, if needed, can treat it at the same time. The use of laparoscopy, however,

has given rise to a number of cases of false negatives in which no ectopic pregnancy was found, but the β-hCG was seen to rise continuously despite an emptied uterus. This should come as no surprise, since, when the ectopic sac diameter is about 5–10 mm, the β-hCG should be about 1000–2000 mIu/ml. This sac should be seen on ultrasound! However, if the β-hCG was lower than 1000 mIu/ml, or if the pregnancy is in the tube but not developing normally, it will often avoid detection even by experienced laparoscopists. Such cases may be treated medically without laparoscopy, using methotrexate and an antimetabolite that has been used extensively to treat gestational trophoblastic diseases. Methotrexate can be given intramuscularly in varying schedules and doses [15, 16].

Culdocentesis

Puncture and aspiration of the cul-de-sac were for many years, probably decades, the gold standard by which to diagnose ruptured ectopic pregnancies. This, indeed, may have been adequate for the times when patients with ectopic pregnancies presented with signs and symptoms or acute pelvic bleeding. Since the introduction of ultrasound in general, and transvaginal ultrasonography in particular, both aided by β-hCG testing, the place of culdocentesis has been taken rightfully by the more accurate and much less invasive imaging technique. A positive culdocentesis, i.e. the finding or aspirating of unclotted blood from the cul-de-sac, indeed is almost pathognomonic for an ectopic pregnancy in a patient with a positive pregnancy test. However, it is extremely important to mention here that transvaginal sonography can determine even the smallest amount of fluid in the cul-de-sac, therefore successfully competing with the more invasive and less accurate test of culdocentesis. It is currently a generally accepted rule that a transvaginal sonographic picture of free pelvic fluid which contains debris-like contents or is of low-level echogenicity in a patient with positive β-hCG and an empty uterus, gives a reliable diagnosis of bleeding ectopic pregnancy.

Vermesh and colleagues [17] suggested that culdocentesis as an invasive and painful procedure has very little real clinical value in diagnosing ectopic pregnancy in a setting where transvaginal sonography and rapid urine or serum pregnancy testing are readily available. This group considers culdocentesis to be of extremely limited value in the diagnostic algorithm of establishing the diagnosis of ectopic pregnancy or ruling it out. If culdocentesis is still required, and transvaginal sonography including a needle-guide to be attached to the shaft of the vaginal probe is available, the use of sonographically-directed transvaginal puncture of the cul-de-sac is advised. In such a fashion, a thin needle can accurately be placed in even the smallest amount of cul-de-sac fluid, avoiding injury of vessels or organs through an otherwise blindly performed procedure.

Since not every emergency room, office or even somewhat larger centers are at present equipped with transvaginal sonography, we agree that the skills of culdocentesis have to be taught in residency programs. However, if the necessity of such resident teaching arises, the procedure should then be performed in the operating room while the patient is under sedation or anesthesia. It should be stressed that a blind puncture of the cul-de-sac may puncture a hollow organ, such as the rectum, blood vessels (resulting in a false-positive test), and it also may not yield blood when blood is indeed present in the cul-de-sac because of the blindly introduced needle tip being in the wrong compartment. We also have to stress the fact that the mere presence of blood aspirated through the puncture of the cul-de-sac may originate from ruptured corpus luteum and not from an ectopic pregnancy which is ruptured. Transvaginal sonography avoids misdiagnosis and, in addition to diagnosing the presence or absence of pelvic fluid, it can easily detect the presence or the absence of intrauterine pregnancy and of adnexal findings as will be shown below.

Ultrasonography

During the last decade, ultrasonography has become the gold standard in the laboratory work-up of patients suspected of ectopic pregnancy. As with almost all areas of gynecology and obstetrics, transabdominal sonography was the first to be employed in scanning the patients suspected of

ectopic pregnancies. The transabdominal evaluation of the patients has a relatively low sensitivity, specifically and positive predictive value. After a short period during which discussions developed as far as the importance of the newly introduced transvaginal technique, transvaginal sonography became the test of choice to work-up the patient suspected of ectopic gestation[18–20]. Despite the fact that in a minority of cases transabdominal sonography is the scanning method through which some ectopic pregnancies located in the most unusual places have been found, transvaginal sonography is the first-line scanning method to establish the diagnosis or to rule it out.

The clinical value of transvaginal sonography in the work-up of patients suspected of ectopic pregnancies is well-supported by the literature[18–22].

If a patient presents with a full bladder, transabdominal sonography can or should be performed first. This can may be advantageous since, if an active intrauterine, or a definite live extrauterine, pregnancy is seen, then a transvaginal scan is probably redundant. Also a transabdominal scan may provide the examiner with a panoramic picture of the pelvis which can guide the transvaginal probe to generate a targeted and clear picture somewhat faster. However, if the patient has an empty bladder, transvaginal sonography should not be delayed and should be the first to be performed. The patient has to be advised not to drink fluids or eat, because she may have to undergo general anesthesia.

A bimanual palpatory examination should precede the transvaginal ultrasound scan to enable comparison of the structures felt by this examination and those obtained with the transvaginal ultrasound scanning.

The transvaginal scanning technique, in general, is described in textbooks of ultrasonography[23,24]. In short, a very compulsive and rigid scanning schedule should be followed. The scanning for a suspected ectopic pregnancy should concentrate first upon the uterus and its cavity with the lining endometrium, extending the attention to both cornual areas, and, even more importantly, the cervical area of the uterus. It is most frustrating if a long scanning time is dedicated to the uterus, adnexa, cul-de-sac, etc., and because of an oversight, a cervical pregnancy is not diagnosed.

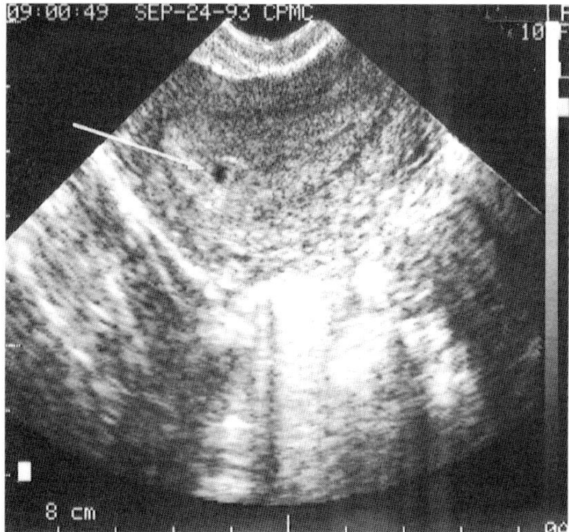

Figure 1 An intrauterine pregnancy at 4 weeks and 1 day from last menstrual period is shown. The gestational sac is embedded in the posterior wall of the endometrium (arrow). The cavity line is clearly seen

Because of its rarity, it is very unlikely that a 'second chance' will be given to 'straighten out' a passed up or missed diagnosis of a cervical pregnancy during the entire professional lifetime of the examiner. After scanning the uterus, the adnexa on both sides should be scanned. An abdominal helping hand to manipulate the pelvic contents can be used. This will be of great help and will give the examiner the feeling of a true manual palpatory pelvic examination. The last to be examined is the cul-de-sac; the tip of the probe should be aimed almost vertically towards the floor to be able to image the cul-de-sac and scrutinize its contents. Touching and exerting gently push–pull motions with the tip of the probe enable the examiner to test for pain and see at the same time where such pain is localized if indeed it is present.

The uterus

As said before, the uterine cavity should be examined first. The uterine cavity may contain one of five distinct findings:

(1) A normal early intrauterine pregnancy (Figure 1);

(2) An abnormal, non-developing, non-live intrauterine pregnancy;

(3) A perfectly well-defined hyperechoic endometrium, which in the presence of a positive pregnancy test is usually considered to be decidua (Figure 2);

(4) Shifting fluid in the cavity (Figure 3), termed 'pseudogestational sac of ectopic pregnancy' (this definition was coined using transbdominal ultrasound); and finally

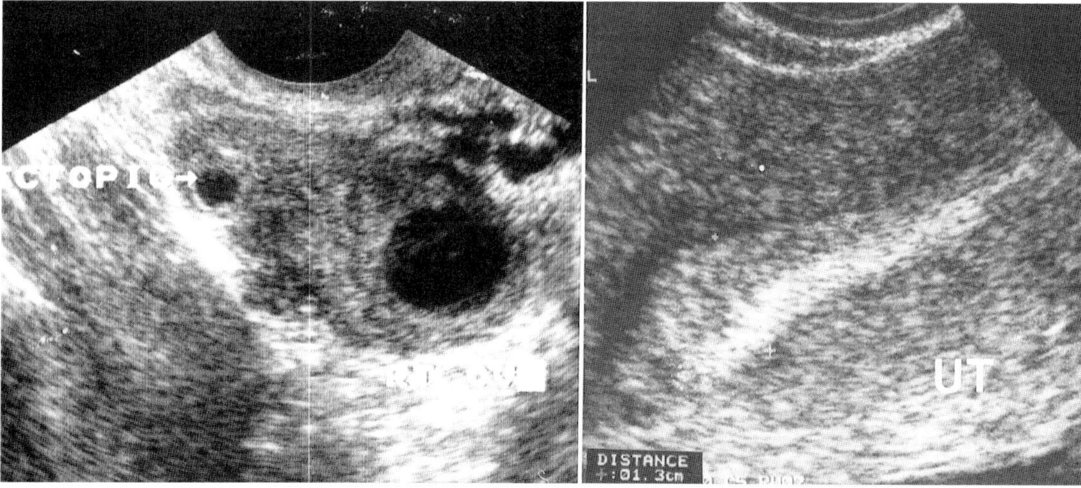

Figure 2 A small and early left tubal ectopic pregnancy imaged together with a corpus luteum at 4 postmenstrual weeks and 5 days (left). The empty uterus (UT) with hyperechoic endometrium (decidual reaction) measuring 1.3 cm is also depicted (right)

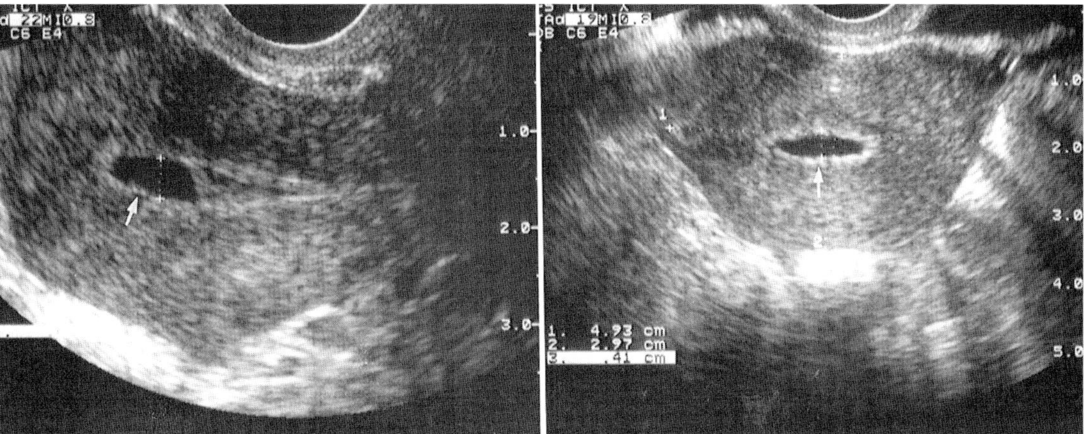

Figure 3 These pictures show the central, intracavitary intrauterine pseudogestational sac (fluid) of a patient with proven ectopic pregnancy at 7 postmenstrual weeks. Note the thin endometrium which is the result of shedding decidual layer (arrow)

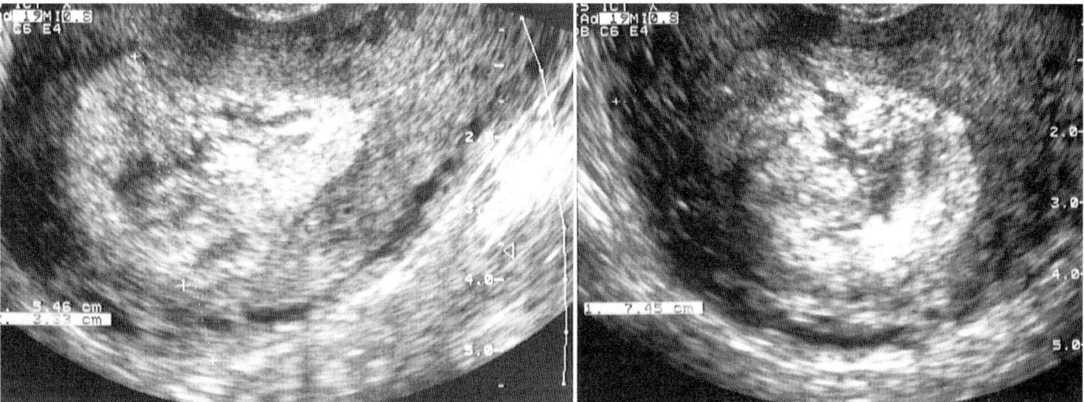

Figure 4 A longitudinal (left) and cross-section (right) of a uterus containing residual products of a conceptus; this time from a known pregnancy failure. At times such as endocavitary transvaginal sonographic picture may raise the differential diagnostic problem of failure of an intrauterine pregnancy and that of a decidual reaction. Curettage and examination of the tissue should be decisive in these cases

(5) Heterogeneous undefined contents (Figure 4) (e.g. the residua of a failed intrauterine pregnancy).

The first three findings are important *diagnostic* findings since they are contributory and clear. The last two intracavitary findings are in reality not very helpful in making a firm diagnosis and therefore are *non-diagnostic*.

Diagnosis of a normal or an abnormal pregnancy does not deserve special mention here, except special cases of heterotopic pregnancies which will be mentioned following this.

The *non-diagnostic* endocavitary findings should be discussed since these present the biggest challenge to the examiner. Once heterogeneous and hyperechoic intracavitary findings are revealed in the presence of a positive β-hCG test, this could be interpreted as a decidual reaction, but it can also represent an early pregnancy failure. If no adnexal findings are detected, and there is no cul-de-sac fluid present, a non-diagnostic endocavitary finding permits a continuous transvaginal sonographic follow-up of the patient

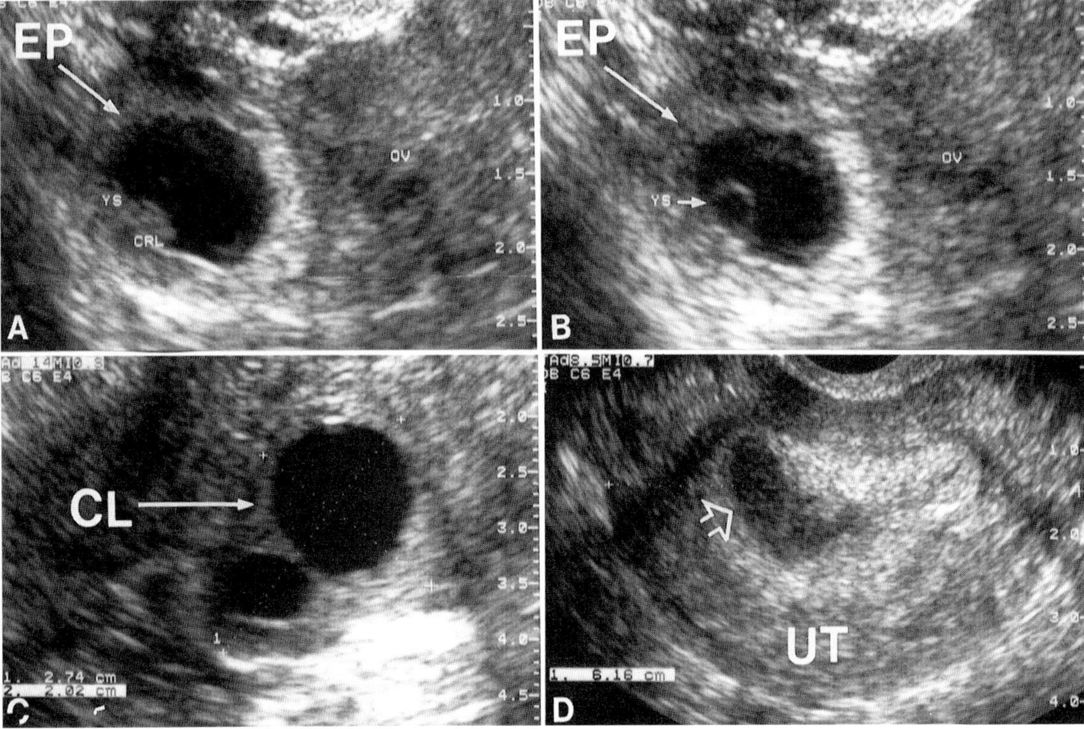

Figure 5 Four sections of ovary, the tube and the uterus of a patient with proven ectopic pregnancy at 6 post-menstrual weeks and 1 day. The ectopic pregnancy (EP) contains the yolk sac (YS) and the fetal pole (CRL). The ipsilateral corpus luteum (CL) is imaged. The uterus (UT) contains a thick decidua as well as sonolucent fluid phase marked by a open arrow. This is the pseudogestational sac of the ectopic pregnancy present in the uterine cavity

followed by serial β-hCG levels. An even better approach is to perform curettage as the next step of the triage.

The *pseudogestational sac*, or in other words a special case of the decidual reaction (Figure 3), has to be given special attention. As far as we are concerned, the definition of the pseudogestational sac is: a sonolucency which is seen along the cavity line, with the endometrial lining symmetrically placed between them; no hyperechoic double-ring can be seen around its irregularly shaped sonolucency (Figure 5D); its shape and location may change during the same or close subsequent examinations; no embryonic or extraembryonic structures are seen within this structure; at times amorphous material is detected amidst it. If color flow is employed, the typical flow within and around the trophoblast of a normal intrauterine pregnancy is not seen.

In contrast, a true intrauterine pregnancy is buried within the endometrium on either side of it and of the cavity line (Figure 1); there is a double hyperechoic ring seen around the gestational sac; its shape is steady and so is its location; in a normal pregnancy, after 5 postmenstrual weeks, embryonic and extraembryonic structures can be seen, and finally, if color is employed, the typical hot flow or low resistance-to-flow pattern is seen in the findings.

At times, color flow sonography may help to distinguish between the true intrauterine pregnancy and the pseudogestational sac[25].

The adnexa

Since most ectopic pregnancies are located within one or the other adnexa, their careful sonographic scanning is the most important part of the transvaginal sonographic evaluation. The most convincing or definitive adnexal finding and the easiest to diagnose is a clear tubal ring consisting

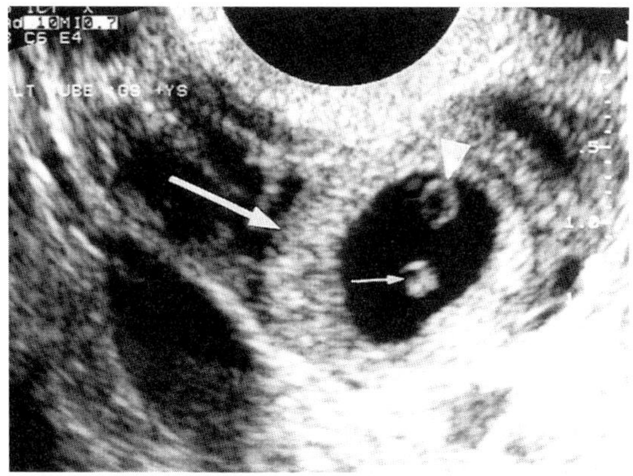

Figure 6 The hyperechoic tubal ring, marked by a long white arrow, at 6 postmenstrual weeks and 1 day. A tubal ectopic pregnancy is shown. The sonolucent sac contains the fetal pole marked by a small white arrow. The fetal pole also demonstrated the embryonic heart beat. The yolk sac is marked by a white arrowhead

of hyperechoic trophoblast, which contains the yolk sac and/or an embryo (Figure 5). The early detection of a live extrauterine gestation is dependent upon the patient population, its awareness of an early booking examination and the proper education of those patients who are at high risk of having an ectopic pregnancy. Various publications in the literature report that ectopic pregnancies with embryonic heart beats come to the attention of obstetricians and gynecologists at a rate of 14–28% of the time[20–22]. There is now very little doubt that transvaginal sonography outperforms transabdominal sonography in finding even the earliest appearing embryonic heart beats in an ectopic location.

There are about 15–20% of ectopic pregnancies which demonstrate what we consider a normal doubling time of the β-hCG levels. Given this fact, one has to assume that these ectopic pregnancies show a normal time sequence in the development of the embryonic and extraembryonic structures. It is therefore also understandable that an early ectopic pregnancy, about 5 postmenstrual weeks, should not yet demonstrate embryonic heart beats, much like its intrauterine counterpart. However, if the ectopic pregnancy reaches 6, 7 or 8 postmenstrual weeks and the ectopic embryo develops normally, the embryonic/extraembryonic structural unit should be identical to the same structural

unit developing within the intrauterine cavity (Figure 6).

Several years ago, we reported on the sequential appearance of extraembryonic and embryonic structures in the normally developing intrauterine pregnancy[26]. Based on this work, the normally developing intrauterine pregnancy can be assessed by relying on the structures present. A normal intrauterine pregnancy of 5 postmenstrual weeks shows a chorionic sac and a yolk sac only; no fetal pole is yet seen. At 6 weeks the fetal pole, and within it embryonic heart beats, can be located. At 7 postmenstrual weeks, the head contains a monolocular sonolucency which is the ventricular system in the embryonic brain. At 8 weeks the physiological midgut hernia is seen[27] and the size of the head equals that of the yolk sac. At 9 postmenstrual weeks, the falx is detectable by vaginal sonography. If we translate this into the embryo developing in an ectopic location, the age of that ectopic embryo can be ascertained in a similar fashion. A well-dated normal pregnancy, regardless of its location, should contain all structural features of the developing embryo. The only significant difference between the extrauterine and intrauterine locations is that the normally developing intrauterine pregnancy is surrounded by myometrium while that developing outside the uterine cavity has no myometrium (in the case of a tubal ectopic pregnancy) or has an extremely thin myometrial layer and is 'tucked' in the corner of the uterus (cornual ectopic pregnancy). The only ectopic pregnancy that is surrounded by muscle layers is the cervical pregnancy; however, that is probably detected quite easily due to its unusual location.

About 85% of ectopic pregnancies are found on the same side as the corpus luteum[28]. One of the most difficult problems in making the correct diagnosis of an ectopic pregnancy is to differentiate between the ectopic pregnancy and the adjacent or contralateral corpus luteum. This task at times appears to be extremely difficult to perform.

The unruptured tubal ring containing trophoblast with or without embryonic and extraembryonic structures, appears to be more echogenic than the texture and echogenicity of the corpus luteum (Figures 7–10). If they happen to be close to each other, this comparison is quite

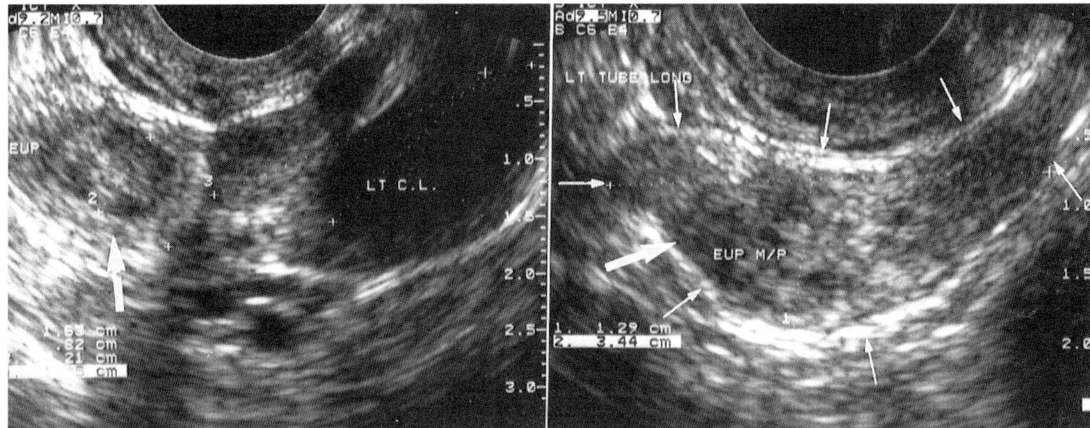

Figure 7 This is an early ectopic pregnancy (arrow) at 6 postmenstrual weeks and 4 days. (Left) the cross-section of the tube imaged side by side with a corpus luteum; (right) the entire ampullar length of the tube containing the ectopic gestation is imaged (small arrows). No heart beat nor embryonic and extraembryonic structures were seen. This was an early demise of an ectopic embryo

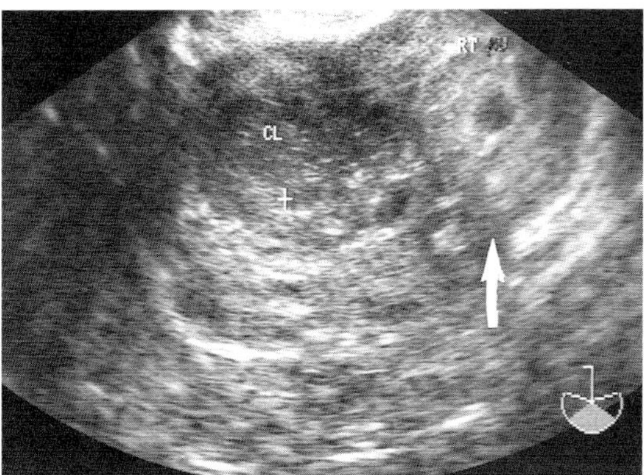

Figure 8 A side-by-side image of a right tubal ectopic pregnancy (white arrow) and the ipsilateral corpus luteum (CL). Note that the corpus luteum is less echogenic than the slightly hyperechoic tubal gestation

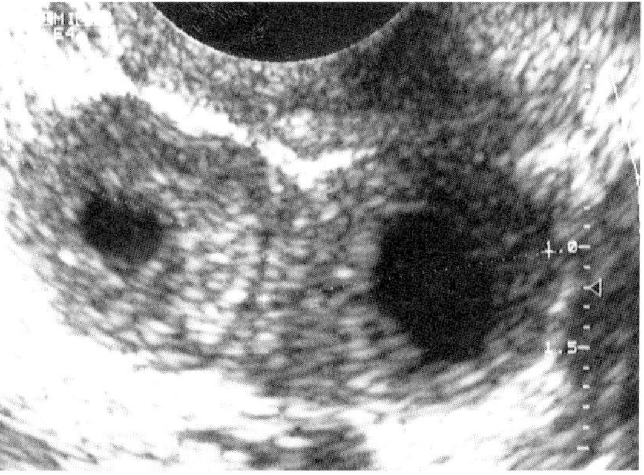

Figure 9 Side-by-side imaging of hyperechoic tubal ring and an ipsilateral corpus luteum showing much less echogenicity

easy, since their echogenicity is, in the overwhelming majority of instances, different. The problem arises in the 15% of ectopic pregnancies located on the contralateral side. One of the small 'tricks' that can be employed is to split the screen and freeze the corpus luteum found on one side and then turn to the ectopic pregnancy located on the contralateral side and freeze it, side by side with the corpus luteum, without touching any of the other controls on the panel. This should be of help in deciding which one of the two structures is more echogenic and is therefore the ectopic gestation.

Another differential diagnostic problem arises

in patients undergoing artificial reproductive technologies or just hormal induction of superovulation. These patients are at high risk for ectopic pregnancies. The large number of 'artificial' corpora lutea resembling the tubal ring of an ectopic pregnancy (Figure 11) is a challenge for even the most experienced sonologist/sonographer.

Brown and Dubilet[29] dealt in depth with the possibility of making the diagnosis of ectopic pregnancy and they analyze the sonographic criteria available for the diagnosis. They came to the conclusion that, as sonographic criteria for ectopic pregnancy become less stringent, the

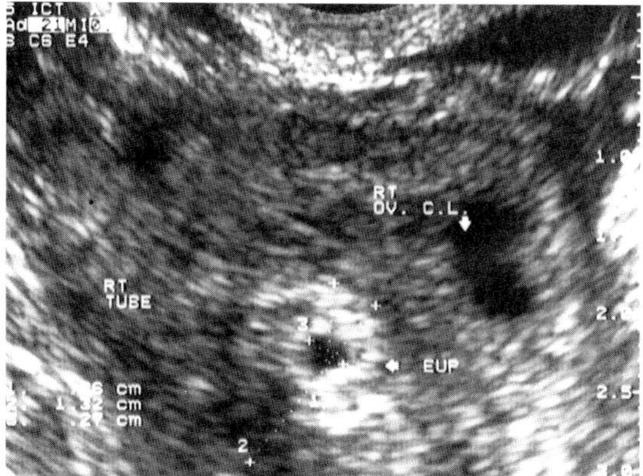

Figure 10 The side-by-side image of a hyperechoic tubal ring of an ectopic pregnancy (EUP) at 4 weeks and 3 days from last menstrual period and the less echoic corpus luteum (CL) in the right ovary (RT OV)

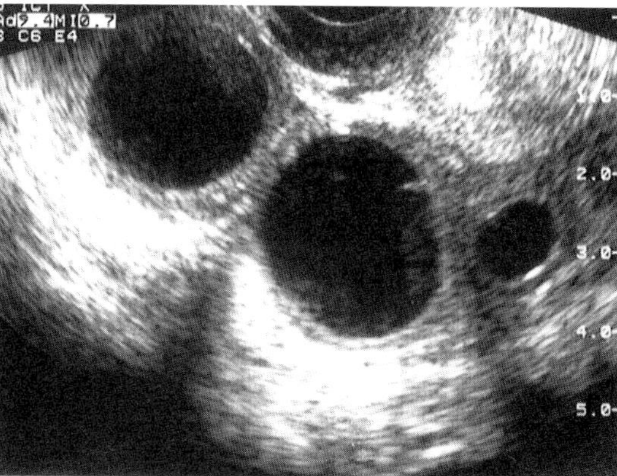

Figure 11 This picture depicts three to four follicles within the ovary filled with sonolucent content. The patient received hormonal enhancement of ovulation. The image is presented to emphasize the differential diagnostic problem. Several of the tubal rings containing sonolucent blood and/or embryonic structures or extraembryonic structures may appear similar to one of these round follicles

sensitivity increases, the specificity decreases and the positive predictive value decreases. According to their study, the likelihood of making the diagnosis of ectopic pregnancy remains greater than 90% even when the adnexal lesion contains no sonographically visible embryo or yolk sac. The likelihood of an ectopic pregnancy is about 95% if a tubal ring is seen in the adnexa and it reaches 100% if an extrauterine embryo with cardiac activity or adnexal fluid collection with yolk sac or an apparent embryo with heart beat are seen.

One has to consider different maneuvers in order to arrive at the correct diagnosis. The first, and maybe the most important, maneuver is to place a helping hand on the anterior abdominal wall of the patient, and use the transvaginal probe as an extension of our examining palpating finger. This combined examination, in conjunction with the picture created on the screen, may be of significant help. Similarly, the probing tip of the transducer touching and pushing different structures may arrive at the point of maximum tenderness which can be located by its shape, location and sonographic structure seen on the screen.

Cul-de-sac

The findings of the cul-de-sac, as far as ectopic pregnancy is concerned, are so important that,

immediately after an empty uterus has been diagnosed, it is worth turning *immediately* to the cul-de-sac and evaluating its content. If it contains fluid (i.e. blood) in larger quantities, then attention should turn to establishing the diagnosis of a ruptured ectopic pregnancy or a tubal abortion in progress. In this case, the patient may need immediate attention. If the cul-de-sac does not contain blood, one can proceed with a lengthy and patient search for the possible ectopic gestation. Patients with perfectly normal intrauterine gestations may show a small or a certain amount of free pelvic fluid. This is particularly true in patients who had ovarian hormonal hyperstimulation and/or egg retrieval. However, the detection of pelvic fluid in increasing quantities significantly enhances the chances of an ectopic pregnancy. The literature reports on about 10–30% of ectopic pregnancies demonstrating fluid in the cul-de-sac[22,30–33].

If, however, no fluid is seen, one can continue with the sonographic and hormonal evaluation of the patient and take the necessary time to arrive at the correct diagnosis.

From a clinical standpoint, there are several important and practical aspects of the presence or the absence of fluid in the cul-de-sac detected by transvaginal sonography.

(1) The more fluid is seen, the more increased the chance of finding a bleeding ectopic pregnancy;

(2) The chances for a ruptured ectopic pregnancy or for a tubal abortion are zero if absolutely no pelvic fluid is found;

(3) An extremely large amount of fluid which coats the uterus from behind and both the right and left sides, making the anchoring ligaments visible, or even extending into the Morrison's pouch (between the liver and the right kidney) signifies a severely bleeding ectopic pregnancy. A small amount of fluid, in contrast, is not helpful since it may result from a leaking corpus luteum, from a slowly bleeding tubal abortion or even the very first stages of an active bleeding. In this case, one should prolong the observational time or rescan the patient within 10–20 min. Transvaginal sonography is not a replacement for regularly checking the vital signs of the patient;

(4) The most important statement regarding fluid in the cul-de-sac is the following: transvaginal sonography is reliable enough to find and to demonstrate pelvic fluid; *therefore, culdocentesis is redundant*;

(5) It is possible to evaluate the echogenicity of the fluid by gently touching and moving the fluid and at the same time increasing the gain settings to observe the swirling motion of the particulate matter in the fluid. Typical echogenicity of the fluid is seen in the right clinical setting of a patient suspected of ectopic pregnancy. It is extremely unlikely that this fluid should be other than blood.

It is possible to estimate the correct amount of fluid in the cul-de-sac. If fluid is detected only below the uterus and in the cul-de-sac, the dimensions of the fluid pocket should be measured in the three cardinal directions, and then the following formula can be used: Volume = $A \times B \times C \times 0.523$ ml. It is also possible to estimate the approximate amount of blood in the pelvis by *gestalt*. If the fluid is only below the uterus in the

cul-de-sac and not extending on the two sides of the uterus and above it, the possible amount is about 50–100 ml. If the blood extends on the two sides of the broad ligament and the fundus, but does not appear in the Morrison's pouch, the amount is between 100 and 200 ml. If fluid is seen to penetrate between the right kidney and the liver, i.e. the Morrison's pouch, it is believed that the amount is exceeding 500 ml. At times, by exerting a push–pull motion on the area of the fluid, bizarre structures are seen to move back and forth. These irregularly shaped somewhat more echogenic structures are the blood clots.

There is a different aspect of examining the cul-de-sac: the blood that collects in this lowest portion of the abdominal–pelvic cavity may result from tubal abortion or tubal rupture. It is extremely important to be able to differentiate between the two. Tubal rupture is a dramatic occurrence associated with pain and changes in the patient's vital signs and a rapid increase in the amount of blood in the cul-de-sac. There is very little that transvaginal sonography or sonography in general can add to the diagnosis of this development. Once the large amount of blood is detected in the cul-de-sac, the patient is better off securing surgical care. However, there is quite a lot to say about the role of transvaginal sonography in diagnosing and managing tubal abortion. Tubal abortion occurs as a result of separation of the products of conception from the site of implantation. As a result of this, these products of conception are expelled or aborted through the fimbrial end of the Fallopian tube. This process is associated at times with slow and other times with quite fast blood flow through the fimbria into the pelvic cavity. If the fimbriated end of the Fallopian tube is constricted, the tube may distend and create a hematosalpinx. If, however, a tubal abortion takes place, a variable amount of blood can gather in the cul-de-sac. The amount of this bleeding need not necessarily be of critical quantities. One has to compare the tubal abortion with that occurring naturally from the uterine cavity. The process of an early pregnancy failure and the process of the uterus expelling the products of conception occurs every day.

The practical conclusion of this is to be able to assess the amount of blood collecting in the cul-de-sac and make a judgement about the dynamics of this process. If the patient is symptomatic (most patients having blood in the cul-de-sac are), and the amount of blood is small, the patient does not necessitate surgical intervention, and should be reassured and the process of tubal abortion and future reabsorption of the blood explained. When treatment other than surgical is performed (e.g. laparoscopic or transvaginally directed puncture and injection of the ectopic pregnancy), the patient should be aware of the possibility of a rather late process of tubal abortion. In this case, conservative management should be instituted by just watching the anatomical area and the cul-de-sac, or administering methotrexate in order to facilitate the decrease of the β-hCG production. If tubal abortion, as a result of puncture procedures or just conservative follow-up, occurs and the patient is symptomatic, *this does not represent failure of the treatment unless significant bleeding is the case.* This process can take place from 3 to 7 or 8 days after the institution of such medical or puncture therapy. It is therefore of practical importance to be able to distinguish between the above-mentioned tubal abortion with slight bleeding and a ruptured ectopic pregnancy or tubal abortion associated with significant amounts of bleeding[34]. The patient's vital signs, levels of hematocrit and, of course, the appearance and quantity of pelvic fluid assessed by transvaginal sonography are imperative.

OTHER SITES OF IMPLANTATION

About 5% of ectopic pregnancies implant in places other than the Fallopian tubes. These, however, present an increased diagnostic challenge. In addition to the difficulty of their exact location, these ectopic pregnancies may bleed more severely and are associated with more morbidity and mortality than the tubal pregnancies[35].

In spite of the fact that heterotopic pregnancy can involve sites other than the Fallopian tubes, the vast majority of such occurrences involve the Fallopian tubes and the uterine cavity. The incidence of heterotopic pregnancies involving the Fallopian tube is about one in 30 000 pregnancies.

However, lately this incidence was recalculated and it is believed that it varies between 1 in 10 000 and 1 in 3889[36–38].

Sotrel and colleagues[39] believe that the heterotopic pregnancy rate is about 1 in 1250 to 1 in 3000. In the group of patients treated with ovulation induction, the incidence of ectopic pregnancy is about 3% and the rate of multiple pregnancies is between 10 and 25%. Using this database, the chances for a heterotopic pregnancy were thought to be as high as 1 in 95 to 1 in 122[40,41]. According to a world collaborative report from 1991[42], the ectopic pregnancy rate was found to be 4.5% and the rate for twins and triplets about 25%. Therefore the heterotopic pregnancy rate in patients having artificial reproductive technologies is about 1% with a range of 1 in 35 to 1 in 450[43].

The incidence of heterotopic pregnancies increases with the increasing number of fertilized oocytes transferred, with the increasing number of pelvic infectious disease episodes and previous tubal damage.

The diagnosis is made usually by ultrasonography and/or laparoscopy. The exact division of these two diagnostic modalities in making the diagnosis, and thus to ascertain their importance, is almost impossible. It is obvious that during the last decade transvaginal sonography has taken the leading role as the 'first-line' diagnostic tool to diagnose any kind of ectopic pregnancy. Most cases are diagnosed between 5 and 8 postmenstrual weeks. The peculiar problem in order to arrive at the diagnosis of heterotopic pregnancy is that, if the diagnosis of an intrauterine pregnancy is established, there is a delay in diagnosing the second pregnancy in an ectopic location. Tal and colleagues[44] surveyed the literature and found that, based upon 91 articles, the detection of the heterotopic pregnancy was made at the same time mostly by ultrasound (49.5%), but in some of the cases the final diagnosis was made only during a surgical procedure aimed at investigating the possibility of an additional and ectopic pregnancy. In one-quarter of the cases, the delay was 1–2 weeks and in about 13% this delay was of 3–4 weeks. In 12% the delay was in excess of 5 weeks. The most frequent location of the ectopic pregnancy (based on 44 articles) in the case of heterotopic pregnancies was, of course, the

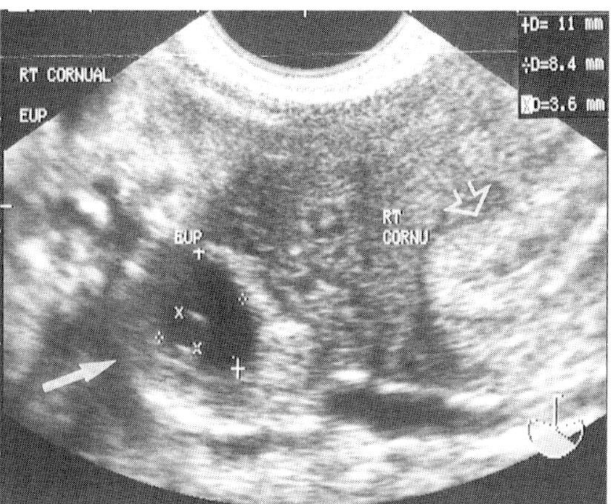

Figure 12 A right cornual ectopic pregnancy (marked by a white arrow) is depicted. The uterus is empty and contains a hyperechoic endometrium (marked by open arrow). The continuity of the endometrial cavity to the ectopic pregnancy in the cornual area is interrupted by normal myometrial tissue. This was a 6 week and 1 day (from last menstrual period) live cornual ectopic pregnancy which was injected with methotrexate

Fallopian tube (about 90%). Cornual implantation occurred in 4.3%.

At this time, we stress the extremely important aspect of diagnosing any ectopic pregnancy but more so the presence of a heterotopic pregnancy. This involves early diagnosis and a high level of suspicion. Special attention has to be given to patients in whom artificial reproductive technologies were involved in achieving the pregnancy or simply if any other high-risk situation is involved. Scanning pregnant patients who underwent ovarian stimulation for ectopic gestation requires skill and time commitment since the sonographic picture may be complicated.

In conclusion, one has to remember that, in the last decade, the incidence of all types of ectopic pregnancies has increased; the incidence of heterotopic pregnancies is no exception!

OTHER SITES OF ECTOPIC GESTATION

For the sake of completeness, cornual, cervical and ovarian pregnancies should be mentioned in spite of the fact that the Fallopian tubes (the subject of this book) are not directly involved. These relatively rare locations are involved

in about 2–3% (combined) of all ectopic pregnancies.

In the case of a *cornual/interstitial pregnancy*, a significant bulge at the cornual area of the uterus is evident by transvaginal sonography. Almost all sonographic features of the tubal ectopic pregnancy apply to the cornual/isthmic pregnancy. A very thin (usually 1–4 mm) myometrial mantle surrounds the typically hyperechoic trophoblastic ring[45–48]. The hyperechoic decidua highlighting the uterine cavity is at least 1 cm remote from the gestational sac (Figure 12).

Ovarian pregnancies are quite difficult to diagnose since the more prevalent tubal pregnancy found in close proximity with the ipsilateral ovary and/or the corpus luteum mimics an ovarian pregnancy quite convincingly[49–51]. If it is impossible to separate the hyperechoic trophoblastic ring from the ovary using the abdominally placed hand and the vaginal transducer in combination, the presence of an ovarian pregnancy can be suspected.

The treatment of the ovarian pregnancy is somewhat different from the treatment of other forms of ectopic gestations. The final diagnosis is made in the pathology laboratory.

Cervical pregnancies are very rare. Only 'stationary' gestational sacs containing a live embryo/fetus in a patient without severe lower abdominal pain should be diagnosed as cervical pregnancies. At least half of the volume of the gestational sac should be found below the imaginary line connecting the two uterine arteries. Color flow studies may present real help in defining such a location of the chorionic sac[52].

At times, different and extremely interesting and bizarre combinations occur as far as the location of ectopic pregnancies is concerned. One of many such combinations is when one Fallopian tube contains two chorionic sacs: twin tubal ectopic pregnancy. Following this a case report is presented to illustrate the diagnostic problem.

CASE REPORT

Case report by Professor Fernando Bonilla-Musoles and Dr Francesco Regata, Department of Obstetrics and Gynecology, University School of Medicine, Valencia, Spain.

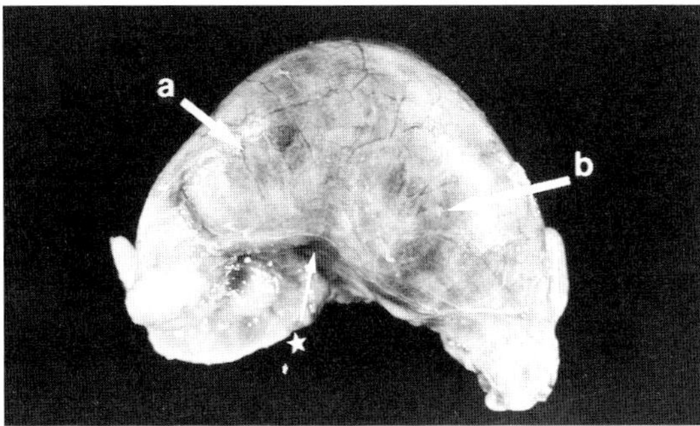

Figure 13 Pathological specimen showing a right Fallopian tube measuring 11×6×5 cm distended into two segments (arrows) which clearly depicted the twin tubal ectopic pregnancy (a, b). Observe the point (star) where the tube is distended into two segments, which was clearly seen by color Doppler (see Color plates 2 and 3)

A 28-year-old woman, gravida 2 para 1 with a last menstrual period of 52 days prior, presented to the emergency room with sudden right lower quadrant pain. She complained of light vaginal bleeding for the past 3 days. Her medical history included an episode of gonorrhea complicated with an episode of acute pelvic inflammatory disease.

The physical examination revealed normal vital signs. The pelvic examination demonstrated a normally sized uterus with a closed cervical os and diffuse pelvic tenderness with a palpable mass in the right adnexa.

Laboratory data included a positive pregnancy test, hemoglobin of 12 g/dl and a hematocrit of 36%.

Transvaginal ultrasound (Aloka SSD 680 EX scanner with a 5-MHz vaginal probe) revealed an empty endometrial cavity with a decidual reaction (Color plate 1). A right adnexal mass was observed, containing two separate well-defined gestational sacs measuring 6 and 8 mm, respectively without embryonic structures (Color plate 2). The area of the suspected tubal pregnancy was examined by color Doppler flow imaging: prominent vascularity was detected between and around both sacs (Color plate 3). Color flow velocity waveform studies revealed low-resistance flows with resistance index (RI) 0.38 and a pulsatility index (PI) 0.45 in the peritrophoblastic area (Color plate 3).

In the right ovary a corpus luteum was present. Color Doppler flow showed a ring of vascularity around the wall with RI, 0.45 and PI, 0.49 typical of an active corpus luteum.

There was a small amount of fluid in the cul-de-sac. The diagnosis of unilateral tubal twin pregnancy was established.

On laparotomy the right tube was observed to be greatly enlarged and distended into two segments (Figure 13). A right salpingectomy was performed.

Pathologic examination of the tube revealed a large number of blood clots, with two independent gestational sacs which corroborated the ultrasound diagnosis. The postoperative course was uncomplicated.

Combined intrauterine and ectopic pregnancy (heterotopic pregnancy) is rare, but the multiple extrauterine pregnancies are exceptional. Isolated reports of multiple ectopic pregnancies can be found in the medical literature.

Etiological factors in ectopic multiple gestations are similar to those seen in single ectopic pregnancies (especially due to an increase in pelvic inflammatory disease and the use of fertility drugs).

Sonography, especially transvaginal sonography, is widely used to evaluate patients in whom ectopic pregnancy is a diagnostic consideration, and so the sonographic diagnostic criteria are well known. However, in our search we have found only three reports of preoperative diagnosis of multiple ectopic pregnancy, two by transabdominal ultrasound and one using transvaginal ultrasound.

Transvaginal color flow Doppler imaging has been instrumental for diagnosing early tubal gestations[13-15].

When the area of the suspected ectopic pregnancy is examined by color flow Doppler imaging, it presents a prominent vascularity, which is regarded as trophoblastic flow. Pulsed Doppler waveform analysis shows a very low impedance signal with resistance index and pulsatility index ranging between 0.30 and 0.48[13-15].

Transvaginal color Doppler ultrasound has improved our knowledge of the hemodynamic alterations involving tubal gestations and is a revolutionary new diagnostic tool in the early detection of tubal pregnancy.

In the presented case, transvaginal color Doppler imaging was a great aid to establish the diagnosis of tubal twin pregnancy preoperatively.

COLOR DOPPLER STUDIES IN ECTOPIC PREGNANCY

Most, if not all, ectopic pregnancies can be diagnosed using gray-scale transvaginal sonography. This statement is important since it reassures all those who own or operate good and reliable gray-scale ultrasound equipment, but do not have color ultrasound.

When color Doppler equipment became available, the technology was used to find blood vessels around the trophoblastic ring and evaluate the flow profile with different quantitative or qualitative measurements. The physiological vascular changes, the scope of which is to supply an increased amount of blood to the implanting blastocyst, are those of a constantly lower and lower impedance and higher velocity flow to the developing placenta. Similar to the increased blood supply to the normal intrauterine pregnancy, physiological vascular changes occur around any ectopic implantation with its developing ectopic trophoblast and placenta.

Even though the pregnancy is implanted outside the uterine cavity, it is rewarding to scan the endometrium and the cavity. Here the lack of findings, typical of a normal intrauterine pregnancy, may be of significance. These negative intra- and pericavitary findings are based on the observation that the swelling decidua and pseudogestational sac do not demonstrate the typical and abundant periplacental and placental trophoblast flow as in an intrauterine gestation. If color flow is detected around a structure resembling an intrauterine pregnancy, flow measurements may be decisive (Figure 14). It has been suggested that velocities below 21 cm/s can be diagnostic for a pseudogestational sac and successfully rule out trophoblastic flow to an interauterine pregnancy (84% sensitivity)[53].

It is important to scan the ovaries carefully. First, the corpus luteum should be localized by gray scale. Color Doppler studies will be able to reveal the typical ring-like, color-rich and low-velocity, low-resistance flow. Finding the corpus luteum enables two assumptions. One assumption is that there may be more changes to help locate the suspected ectopic pregnancy (if it is not easily detected) on the ipsilateral side. Eighty-six per cent of the ectopic pregnancies were found to be on the side of the corpus luteum[54]. The second assumption – true only in cases in which no hormonal superovulation was practiced – that, if a second color-rich ring-like structure is found, it may be consistent with the abundant blood supply of the tubal ring (in the case of a tubal pregnancy). It is important to state here that one should not rely upon the resistance to flow (pulsatility index and resistance index) measurements only, since both the corpus luteum and the flow to any ectopic pregnancy (tubal, cornual or other) will be low and therefore non-discriminatory.

Last but not least, it is important to describe the findings using color Doppler studies within, or around the ectopic pregnancy itself. It seems reasonable to apply 'color interrogation' any time a finding is in doubt and the suspicion of an ectopic gestation still exists (Figure 14). It is very difficult to separate the true additional sensitivity and specificity of this scanning modality over that of the customary gray scale. As said before, gray scale alone yields satisfactory clinical results.

As far as the color Doppler image and the flow measurements are concerned, the following facts can be listed. First, ectopic pregnancies with higher β-hCG levels demonstrate a lower resistance to flow and a higher 'quantity' of color. Second, 'live' or still actively β-hCG-producing ectopic pregnancies show a 'hot' flow pattern in addition to a higher diastolic flow as opposed to ectopic pregnancies in which there is a long-standing embryonic demise ('missed ectopic pregnancy') and in which less flow and higher resistance to flow are seen.

After reviewing the literature and based upon personal experience, it is clear that color Doppler studies are a convenient complement to the high-frequency transvaginal sonographic gray-scale modality in dealing with the diagnosis of ectopic pregnancy. The diagnosis is made faster and more reliably and it is reasonable to say that this is done by a marginally (at times important) improved accuracy. The interested reader is referred to the literature to obtain additional and more detailed information[55–63].

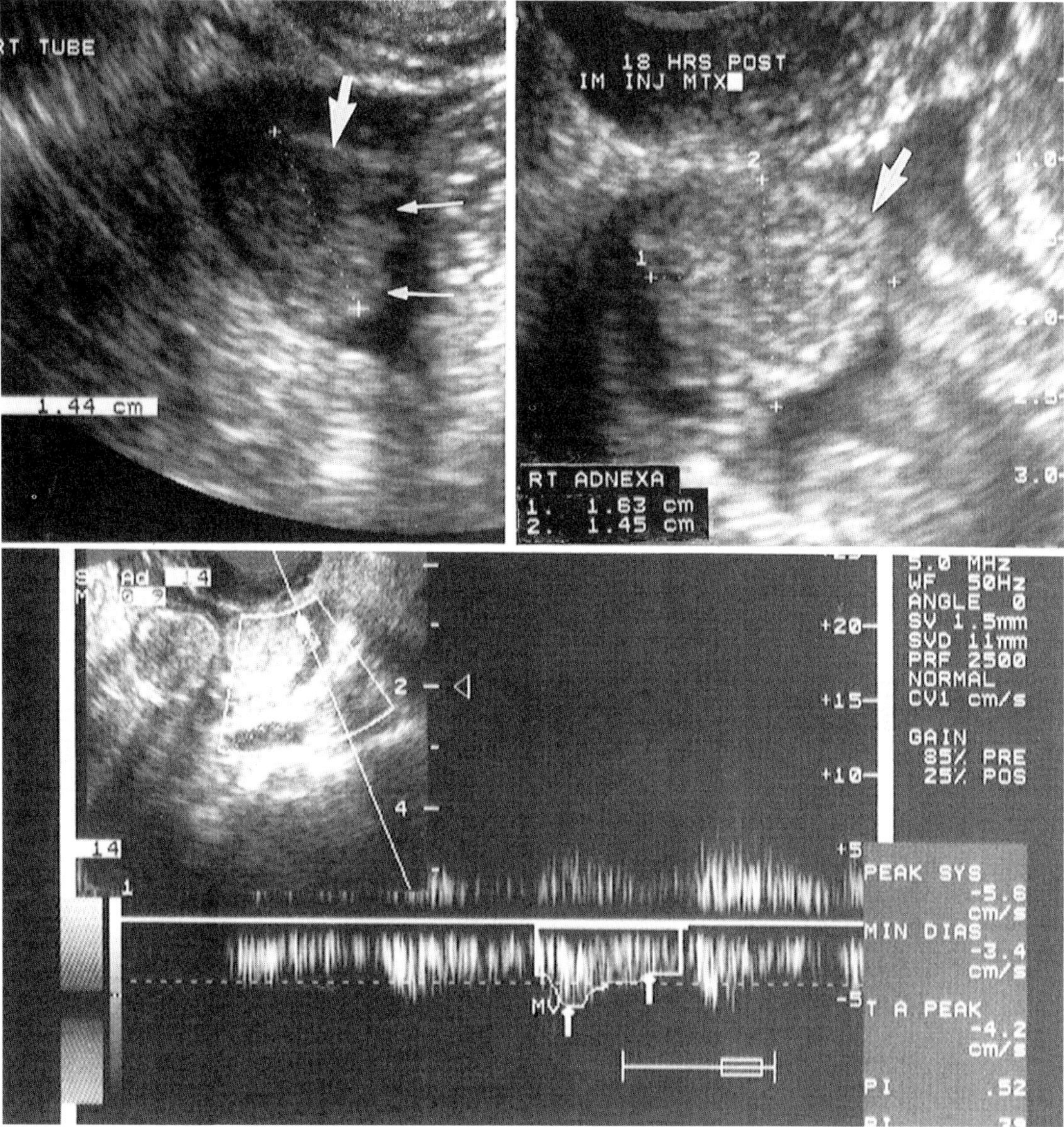

Figure 14 A 5 week 5 days (from last menstrual period) 'missed' ectopic pregnancy is imaged. The fimbria of the left tube is marked by small arrows. The ectopic pregnancy containing probably the blood clot is marked by the large arrow. The dilated tube measures 1.63 × 1.45 cm. Methotrexate injection was administered to this patient 18 hours before this image was taken. The pulsatility index was 0.52 and the resistance index was 0.39

The use of color Doppler studies in cornual and in cervical pregnancies is less documented in the literature. Our experience is that it is most useful in the follow-up of conservatively managed cases or in cases in which the puncture injection of the trophoblastic sac itself or parenteral methotrexate was used[46,52]. In these cases, the qualitative evaluation of the area in question seems to reassure the observer without any confirmatory proof or supportive studies in the literature.

ULTRASOUND–GUIDED PUNCTURE AND INJECTION OF ECTOPIC PREGNANCY

After the diagnosis of a live tubal, cornual, or cervical pregnancy is established, the appropriate way to treat the specific ectopic gestation is selected. It is not in the scope of this chapter to discuss the various well-established or customary treatment modalities of each and every kind or variation of ectopic gestations. We present a specific way to treat the ectopic pregnancy: the use of puncture and injection. The reason for this is that it is performed with transvaginal sonographic guidance. In the hands of several groups, transvaginal puncture procedure and injection of agents such as potassium chloride, methotrexate or glucose is a valid option to be considered.

Even though transvaginal sonography-directed puncture and injection with methotrexate of an ectopic pregnancy was performed and reported 6 years ago, the technique did not spread as fast as expected.

The technique consists of attaching a needle guide to the vaginal probe and puncturing the structure with the thinnest possible needle under sonographic control. When the needle is in place, potassium chloride (2 mEq/ml) or methotrexate solution (25–50 mg in 1 ml) is injected (Figure 15).

After reviewing 136 published cases of punctures[46, 52, 64–81], it became clear that the relatively low success rate (80%) is due to several factors: because of the few cases treated this way in almost every center, the individuals performing the puncture technique are operating still on the lower end of their learning curve. Furthermore, there is a wide variation between the different authors as far as the indications for the procedure, the gestational ages or the maximal size of the lesions at which the puncture treatment is performed.

Obviously it is hard to compare and evaluate critically the usefulness of the puncture treatment. The 'common denominator' so important for a fair comparison between cases is missing. Different kinds of ectopic pregnancies, non-viable embryos, embryos/fetuses of different gestational ages and sizes have been injected with various amounts of dissimilar agents through assorted needle gauges.

Most physicians are unaware of the natural history, the symptoms and signs as well as the ultrasonographic evolution of the postinjection period[34].

Our list of prerequisites to be considered for puncture treatment of any ectopic site hosting a pregnancy are:

(1) Compliant, stable, asymptomatic patient, capable of understanding the advantages and the disadvantages as well as the possible complications of the procedure;

(2) Live, unruptured pregnancy with heart beats, and no active bleeding;

(3) The size of the lesion is 4 cm or less;

(4) The age of the pregnancy is $8\frac{1}{2}$–9 postmenstrual weeks or less;

(5) A 21-gauge needle operated by the automated spring-loaded puncture device (Labotect, Göttingen, Germany[46, 52, 64, 65, 70, 82] (Figure 16);

(6) Signed (Institutional Review Board-approved) informed patient consent.

In our institutions, all of the above-mentioned prerequisites have to be fulfilled.

As far as the postpuncture convalescent period is concerned, all those engaging in such treatment should be familiar with the following. There is a prolonged and slow decline in the levels of β-hCG. Injecting methotrexate instead of potassium chloride shortens the return of the hormonal levels to non-pregnant values[46,52,70,71,76]. Pain and lower abdominal cramping[34] may be caused by the possible tubal abortion into the pelvis with some (but usually not profuse) bleeding. The patient's vital signs and the amount of blood in the cul-de-sac should be monitored. Another reason for this lower abdominal pain may be the passage of the uterine contents (decidual cast). This may occur days later and can be easily diagnosed once the awareness of it exists.

Transvaginal gray-scale and color Doppler findings include a slight increase in size of the injected lesion as well as a slow degenerative process of the yolk sac and the embryonic pole.

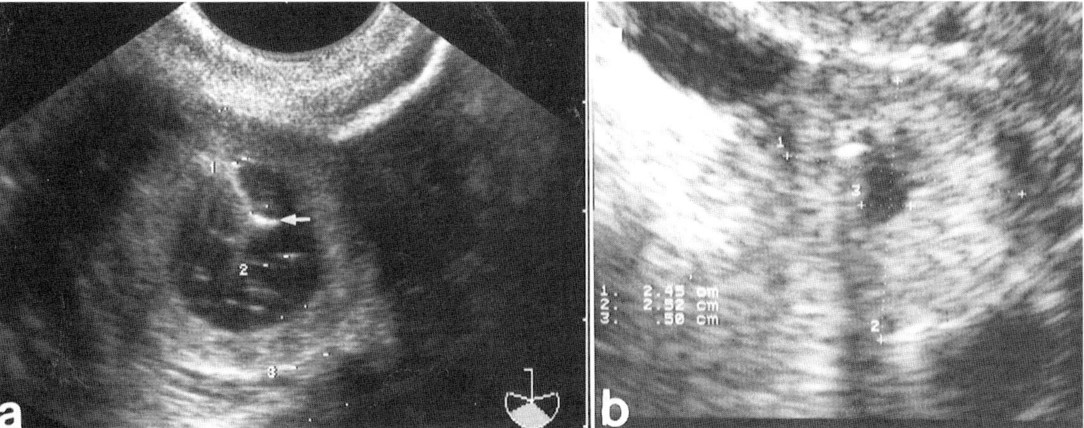

Figure 15 Puncture and injection treatment of tubal ectopic pregnancy. A live 6 week 4 days (from last menstrual period) ectopic pregnancy with a fetal pole of 7.0 mm was injected using the automated puncture device mated to the transvaginal ultrasound probe. (a) The arrow marks the tip of the needle which is in the small embryo to a depth of 1.8 cm. The yolk sac is seen on the left of the needle; 50 mg methotrexate was injected. (b) Twenty hours later the embryonic and extraembryonic structures are no longer seen, the chorionic sac is smaller, the outer diameter of the tube is the same (2.5 cm)

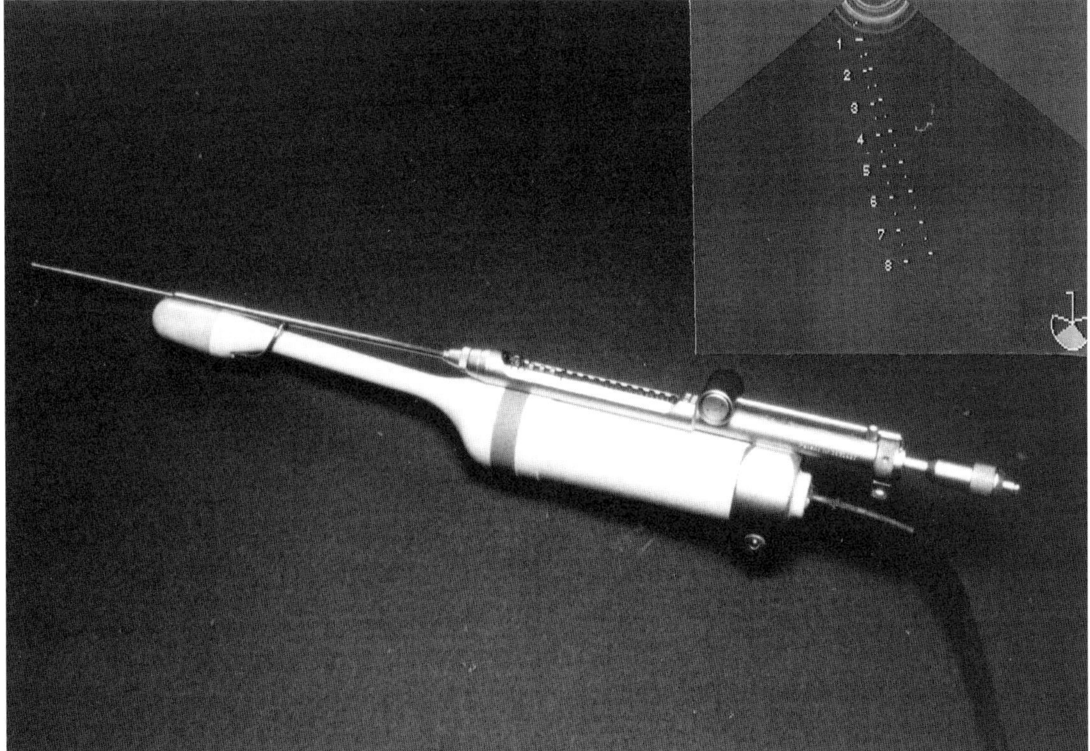

Figure 16 The automated spring-loaded puncture device with a needle (released position) is mated to the transvaginal ultrasound probe. The inlay shows the double, software-generated, direction and depth markers. The depth of the needle can be set by the operator

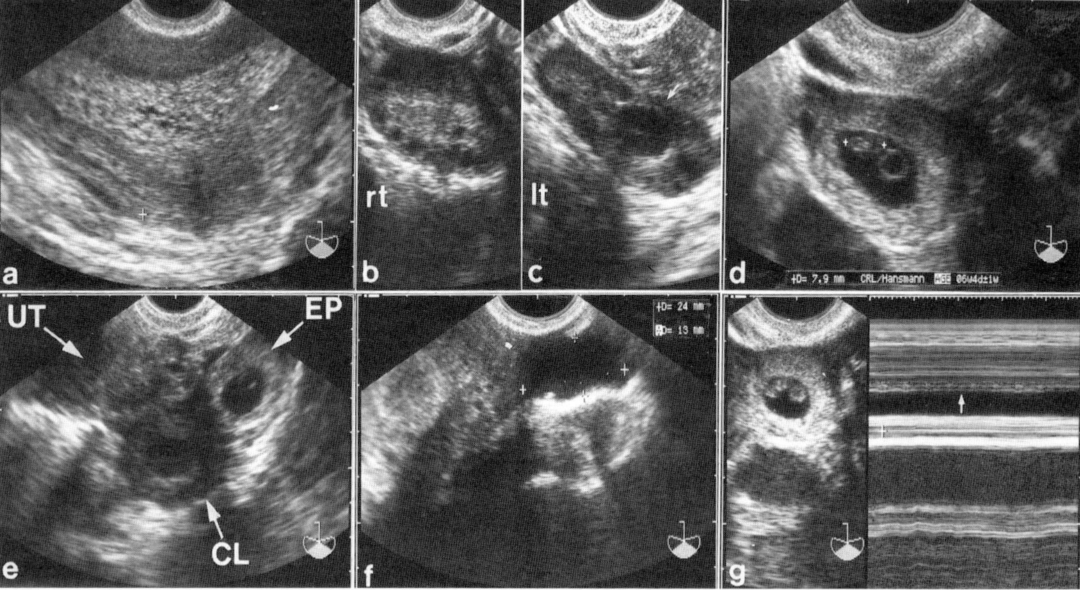

Figure 17 Pictorial description of a transvaginal sonographic work-up of a patient suspected of ectopic pregnancy. (a) Scanning of the uterus reveals a hyperechoic, thick endometrium without an obvious trophoblastic sac; (b and c) right and left ovaries; in the left ovary the corpus luteum is visible (arrow); (d) the tubal ring on the left side measured 2.5 cm in diameter. The yolk sac and the embryonic pole (CRL = 7.9 mm at 6 postmenstrual weeks and 4 days) are seen; (e) this view contains the uterus (UT), left ovary with the corpus luteum (CL) and the more echogenic tubal ring (EP); (f) in the cul-de-sac a small amount of fluid (2.4 × 3 1.3 cm) is seen on the longitudinal section; (g) documentation of the embryonic heart beats (arrow)

Color flow studies reveal an increased quantity of color due to the abundant vascularity and venous spaces.

Our feeling is that salpingocentesis (the injection of the ectopic gestation situated in the Fallopian tube) may not become widely used. However, the injection of cornual pregnancies[46] and of cervical pregnancies[52] has much to offer to patients in terms of a less invasive procedure, which may replace and avoid a more complication-ridden, at times extremely bloody, surgical treatment. This puncture procedure may at times save the patient from hysterotomy with future Cesarean sections or even from losing the entire uterus.

CONCLUSIONS

The introduction of β-hCG testing and transvaginal sonography has changed the diagnostic approach to the patient suspected of ectopic preg-nancy. All this change occurred in the last decade when a real breakthrough to early and accurate detection of this disease became generally available.

It is obvious that the term 'ectopic pregnancy' contains different manifestations of the disease, at various gestational ages, each one with its own variations and sonographic expressions. The only right way to arrive at the diagnosis and the appropriate management plan is to combine the history, clinical signs and symptoms with the readily available transvaginal sonographic picture and level (or the trend) of β-hCG testing. The importance of a conscientious and extremely systematic scanning routine to find or to rule out an ectopic pregnancy (Figure 17) cannot be overstressed.

The ability to bring transvaginal sonography and a fast monoclonal antibody testing of the patient's urine into the gynecologist's office or the emergency room is another step forward to enable a faster detection of earlier and less life-threatening stages of this disease. Transvaginal sonography enables the selection of the adequate and proper as well as the least invasive treatment for the respective kind of ectopic pregnancy.

We are sure that shortening the diagnostic process is advantageous not only to the clinician but also for the patients.

References

1. Centers for Disease Control (1987). Ectopic pregnancy – United States, 1987. *MMWR*, **39**, 401–4

2. Dorfman, S.F., Grimess, D.A., Cates, W. Jr, *et al.* (1984). Ectopic pregnancy mortality. United States, 1979 to 1980: clinical aspects. *Obstet. Gynecol.*, **64**, 386–90

3. Young, P.L., Safteas, A.F., Atrash, H.K., Lawson, H.W. and Petrey, F.F. (1991). National trends in the management of tubal pregnancy, 1970–1987. *Obstet. Gynecol.*, **78**, 749–52

4. Corson, S.K. and Batzer, F.R. (1986). Ectopic pregnancy: a review of the etiologic factors. *J. Reprod. Med.*, **31**, 78

5. Sopelak, V.M. and Bates, G.B. (1987). Role of transmigration and abnormal embryogenesis in ectopic pregnancy. *Clin. Obstet. Gynecol.*, **30**, 210

6. Marchbanks, P.A., Annegers, J.F., Coulam, C.B., Strathy, J.H. and Kurland, L.T. (1988). Risk factors for ectopic pregnancy. A population-based study. *J. Am. Med. Assoc.*, **259**, 1823

7. Kadar, N., DeVore, G. and Romero, R. (1981). Discriminatory hCG zone. Its use in sonographic evaluation for ectopic pregnancy. *Obstet. Gynecol.*, **58**, 156–61

8. Nyberg, D.A., Filly, R.A., Mahoney, B.S. *et al.* (1985). Early gestation: correlation of hCG levels and sonographic identification. *Am. J. Roentgenol*, **144**, 951–4

9. Goldstein, S. (1988). Very early pregnancy detection with endovaginal ultrasound. *Obstet. Gynecol.*, **72**, 200–4

10. Timor-Tritsch, I.E., Rottem, S. and Thaler, I. (1988). Review of transvaginal ultrasonography: a description with clinical application. *Ultrasound Q.*, **6**, 1–32

11. Peisner, D. B., Timor-Tritsch, I.E., Margulis, E. *et al.* (1988). Analysis of beta-hCG and sac size in early pregnancy. *J. Ultrasound Med.*, **7** (Suppl.), 5106

12. Fossum, G.T., Dvajan, V. and Kletzky, D.A. (1988). Early detection of pregnancy with transvaginal ultrasound. *Fertil. Steril.*, **49**, 788–91

13. Bernaschek, G., Ruaelstorfer, R. and Csaicsich, P. (1988). Vaginal sonography versus serum human chorionic gonadotropin in early detection of pregnancy. *Am. J. Obstet. Gynecol.*, **158**, 608–12

14. Stovall, T.G., Ling, F.W., Cope, B.J. and Buster, J.E. (1989). Preventing ruptured ectopic pregnancy utilizing a single serum progesterone. *Am. J. Obstet. Gynecol.*, **160**, 1425–8

15. Stovall, T.G., Ling, F.E.W., and Gray, L. (1991). Single-dose methotrexate for treatment of ectopic pregnancy. *Obstet. Gynecol.*, **77**, 754–7

16. Stovall, T., Ling, F. and Buster, J.E. (1989). Outpatient chemotherapy for unrupted ectopic pregnancy. *Fertil. Steril.*, **51**, 435–8

17. Vermesh, M., Gvaczykowsky, J.W. and Sauer, M.V. (1990). Reevaluation of the culdocentesis in the management of ectopic pregnancy. *Am. J. Obstet. Gynecol.*, **162**, 411–13

18. Timor-Tritsch, I.E. and Rottem, S. (1987). Transvaginal sonographic study of the Fallopian tube. *Obstet. Gynecol.*, **70**, 424–8

19. de Crespigny, I.C. (1988). Demonstration of ectopic pregnancy by transvaginal ultrasound. *Br. J. Obstet Gynaecol.*, **95**, 1253–6

20. Timor-Tritsch, I.E., Yeh, M.N., Peisner, D.B., Lesser, K.B. and Slavik, T.A. (1989). The use of transvaginal ultrasonography in the diagnosis of ectopic pregnancy. *Am. J. Obstet. Gynecol.*, **161**, 157–61

21. Cacciatore, B., Stenman, U-H. and Ylostalo, P. (1989). Comparison of abdominal and vaginal sonography in suspected ectopic pregnancy. *Obstet. Gynecol.*, **73,** 770–4

22. Stiller, R.J., de Regt, R.H. and Blair, E. (1989). Transvaginal ultrasonography in patients at risk for ectopic pregnancy. *Am. J. Obstet. Gynecol.*, **161**, 930–3

23. Rottem, S. and Timor-Tritsch, I.E. (eds.) (1991). *Transvaginal Sonography.* (New York: Chapman and Hall)

24. Goldstein, S.R. and Timor-Tritsch, I.E. (eds.) (1995). *Gynecologic Ultrasound.* pp. 49–54, 169–86. (New York: Churchill and Livingstone)

25. Turetsky, D.B., Alexander, A.A. and Linden, S.S. (1991). Pseudogestational sac of ectopic pregnancy stimulating intrauterine pregnancy with transvaginal sonography. *J. Clin. Ultrasound.* **19**, 120–3

26. Warren, W.B., Timor-Tritsch, I.E., Peisner, D.B., Raju, S. and Rosen, M.G. (1989). Dating of the early pregnancy by sequential appearance of embryonic structures. *Am. J. Obstet. Gynecol.*, **161**, 747–53

27. Timor-Tritsch, I.E., Warren W.B., Peisner, D.B. and Pirrone, E. (1989). First trimester midgut herniation: a high frequency transvaginal sonographic study. *Am. J. Obstet. Gynecol.*, **161**, 831–3

28. Pellerito, J.S., Taylor, K.J.W., Quedens-Case, C. *et al.* (1992). Ectopic pregnancy: evaluation with endovaginal color flow imaging. *Radiology*, **183**, 407–11

29. Brown, D.L. and Doubilet, P.M. (1994). Transvaginal sonography for diagnosing ectopic pregnancy: positivity criteria and performance

characteristics. *J. Ultrasound Med.*, **13**, 259–66

30. Romero, R., Copel, J.A., Kadar, N. *et al.* (1985). Value of culdocentesis in the diagnosis of ectopic pregnancy. *Obstet. Gynecol.*, **65**, 319–22

31. Fleischer, A.C., Pennell, R.G., McKee, M.S. *et al.* (1990). Ectopic pregnancy: features at transvaginal sonography. *Radiology*, **174**, 375–8

32. Timor-Tritsch, I.E., Peisner, D.B. and Monteagudo, A. (1991). Transvaginal sonography in the diagnosis of ectopic pregnancy. In Grünfeld, L. (ed.) *Ultrasonography in Reproductive Medicine. Infert. Reprod. Med. Clin. N. Am.*, **2**, 727–39

33. Rottem, S., Thaler, I. and Timor-Tritsch, I.E. (1991). Classification of tubal gestation by transvaginal sonography. *Ultrasound Obstet. Gynecol.*, **1**, 197

34. Carson, S.A., and Buster, J.E. (1993). Ectopic pregnancy. *N. Engl. J. Med.*, **329**, 1174–81

35. Bayless, R.B. (1987). Nontubal ectopic pregnancy. *Clin. Obstet. Gynecol.*, **30**, 191–9

36. Reece, E.A., Petrie, R.H., Sirmans, M.F., Finster, M. and Todd, W.D. (1983). Combined intrauterine and extrauterine gestations: a review. *Am. J. Obstet. Gynecol.*, **146**, 323

37. Richards, S.R., Stempel, L.E. and Carlton, B.H. (1982). Heterotopic pregnancy: re-appraisal of incidence. *Am. J. Obstet. Gynecol.*, **142**, 928–30

38. Bello, G.V., Schonholz, D., Moshirpur, J., Jeng, D-Y. and Berkowitz, R.L. (1986). Combined pregnancy: The Mount Sinai experience. *Obstet. Gynecol. Surv.*, **41**, 603–13

39. Sotrel, G., Rao, R. and Scommegma, A. (1976). Heterotopic pregnancy following Clomid treatment. *J. Reprod. Med.*, **16**, 78–80

40. Gemzell, C., Guillome, J. and Wang, C.F. (1982). Ectopic pregnancy following treatment with human gonadotropins. *Am. J. Obstet. Gynecol.*, **143**, 761–5

41. Berger, M.J. and Taymor, M.L. (1972). Simultaneous intrauterine and tubal pregnancies following ovulation induction. *Am. J. Obstet. Gynecol.*, **113**, 812–13

42. Goldman, G.A., Fisch, B., Ovadia, J. and Tadir, Y. (1992). Heterotopic pregnancy after assisted reproductive technologies. *Obstet. Gynecol. Surv.*, **47**, 217–21

43. World Collaborative Report (1993). Presented at the *VIIIth World Congress on In Vitro Fertilization and Alternate Assisted Reproduction*, Kyoto, Japan, Sept. 12–15

44. Tal, J., Hadad, S., Gordon, N. and Timor-Tritsch, I.E. (1995). Heterotopic pregnancy after ovulation induction and assisted reproductive technologies: a literature review from 1971 to 1973. *Fertil. Steril.*, in press

45. Sherer, D.M., Allen, T., Singh, G.S. and Wods, J.R. Jr. (1990). Transvaginal sonographic diagnosis of an unruptured interstitial pregnancy. *J. Clin. Ultrasound*, **18**, 582–5

46. Timor-Tritsch, I.E., Monteagudo, A., Matera, C. and Veit, C.R., (1992). Sonographic evaluation of cornual pregnancies treated without surgery. *Obstet.*

Gynecol., **79**, 1044–9

47. Oelsner, G.G., Admon, D., Shalev, E., Shaler, J., Kukin, E. and Mashiach, S. (1993). A new approach for the treatment of interstitial pregnancy. *Fertil. Steril.*, **59**, 924–5

48. Shalev, E., Romano, S. and Bustan, M. (1989). Interstitial pregnancy – successful treatment with methotrexate. *Isr. J. Med. Sci.*, **25**, 239–40

49. Grimes, H.G., Nosal, R.A. and Gallagher, J.C. (1983). Ovarian pregnancy: a series of 24 cases. *Obstet. Gynecol.*, **61**, 174

50. Athey, P.A., Jayson, H.T., Estrada, R. and Watson, A.B. Jr (1990). Sonographic findings in primary ovarian pregnancy. *J. Clin. Ultrasound*, **18**, 730–2

51. Malinger, G., Achiron, R., Treschan, O. and Zakut, H. (1988). Ovarian pregnancy – ultrasonographic diagnosis. *Acta Obstet. Gynecol. Scand.*, **67**, 561–3

52. Timor-Tritsch, I.E., Monteagudo, A., Mandeville, E.O., Peisner, D.B., Anaya-Parra, G. and Pirrone, E.C. (1994). Successful management of viable cervical pregnancy by local injection of methotrexate guided by transvaginal sonography. *Am. J. Obstet. Gynecol.*, **170**, 737–9

53. Dillon, E.H., Feycock, A.L. and Taylor, K.J.W. (1990). Pseudogestational sacs: Doppler US differentiation from normal or abnormal intrauterine pregnancies. *Radiology*, **176**, 359–64

54. Pellerito, J.S., Taylor K.J.W., Quadens-Case, C., Hammers, L.W., Scoutt, L.M., Ramos, I.M. and Meyer W.R. (1992). Ectopic pregnancy: evolution with endovaginal color flow imaging. *Radiology*, **183**, 407–11

55. Taylor, K.J.W., Ramos, I.M., Feycock, A.L. *et al.* (1989). Ectopic pregnancy duplex Doppler evaluation. *Radiology*, **173**, 93–6

56. Taylor, K.J.W. and Meyer W.R. (1991). New technologies in the diagnosis of ectopic pregnancy. *Obstet. Gynecol. Clin. North. Am.*, **18**, 39–54

57. Emerson, D.S., Cartier, M.S., Altieri, L.A. *et al.* (1992). Diagnostic efficacy of endovaginal color Doppler flow imaging in an ectopic pregnancy screening program. *Radiology*, **183**, 413–20

58. Jurkovic, D., Bourne, T.H., Jauniaux, E. *et al.* (1992). Transvaginal color Doppler study of blood flow in ectopic pregnancies. *Fertil. Steril.*, **57**, 68–73

59. Kirchler, H.C., Kolle, D. and Schwegel, P. (1988). Changes in tubal blood flow in evaluating ectopic pregnancy. *Ultrasound Obstet. Gynecol.*, **2**, 283–8

60. Tekay, A and Jouppila, P. (1992). Color Doppler flow as an indicator of trophoblastic activity in tubal pregnancies detected by transvaginal ultrasound. *Obstet. Gynecol.*, **80**, 995–9

61. Kurjak, A., Zalud, I. and Volpe, G. (1990) Conventional B-mode and transvaginal color Doppler in ultrasound assessment of ectopic pregnancy. *Acta Med. Jugosl.*, **44**, 91–103

62. Atri, M. (1993). Ectropic pregnancy: evaluation with endovaginal color Doppler flow imaging. *Radiology*, **187**, 19

63. Brown, D.L. (1993). Diagnosis of ectopic pregnancy

with endovaginal color Doppler US. *Radiology*, **187**, 20–4

64. Feichtinger, W. and Kemeter, P. (1987). Conservative treatment of ectopic pregnancy by transvaginal aspiration under sonographic control and methotrexate injection. *Lancet*, **1**, 381

65. Feichtinger, W. and Kemeter, P. (1989), Treatment of unruptured ectopic pregnancy by needling of sac and injection of methotrexate or PGE2 under transvaginal sonography control: report of 10 cases. *Arch. Gynecol. Obstet.*, **246**, 85–9

66. Robertson, D.E., Smith, W. and Moye, M.A.H. (1987). Reduction of ectopic pregnancy by injection under ultrasound control. *Lancet*, **1**, 974–5

67. Robertson, D.E., Smith, W. and Craft, I. (1987). Reduction of ectopic pregnancy by ultrasound methods. *Lancet*, **2**, 1524–5

68. Leeton, J. and Davison, G. (1988). Non-surgical management of unruptured tubal pregnancy with intra-amniotic methotrexate: preliminary report of two cases. *Fertil. Steril.*, **50**, 167–9

69. Timor-Tritsch, I.E., Baxi, L. and Peisner, D.B. (1989). Transvaginal salpingocentesis: a new technique for treating ectopic pregnancy. *Am. J. Obstet. Gynecol.*, **160**, 459–61

70. Timor-Tritsch, I.E., Peisner, D.B. and Monteagudo, A. (1991). Puncture procedures utilizing transvaginal ultrasonic guidance. *Ultrasound Obstet. Gynecol.*, **1**, 144–50

71. Menard, A., Crequat, J., Mandelbrot, L., Hauuy, J.P. and Madelanat, P. (1990). Treatment of unruptured tubal pregnancy by local injection of methotrexate under transvaginal sonographic control. *Fertil. Steril.*, **54**, 47–50

72. Aboulghar, M.A., Mansour, R.T. and Serour, G.I. (1990). Transvaginal injection of potassium chloride and methotrexate for the treatment of tubal pregnancy with a live fetus. *Hum. Reprod.*, **5**, 887–8

73. Fernandez, H., Baton, C., Lelaidier, C. and Frydman, R. (1991). Conservative management of ectopic pregnancy: prospective randomized clinical trial of methotrexate versus prostaglandin sulpostrone by combined transvaginal and systemic administration. *Fertil. Steril.*, **55**, 746

74. Tulandi, T., Bret, P.M., Atri, M. and Senterman, M. (1991). Treatment of ectopic pregnancy by transvaginal intratubal methotrexate administration. *Obstet. Gynecol.*, **77**, 627–43

75. Popp, L.W., Mettler, L., Weisner, H., Mecke, I., Freys, I. and Semm, K. (1991). Ectopic pregnancy treatment using pelviscopic or vaginosonographically guided intrachorionic injection of methotrexate. *Ultrasound Obstet. Gynecol.*, **1**, 136–43

76. Shalev, E., Zalel, Y., Bustan, M. and Weiner, E. (1991). Ectopic pregnancy: sonographically guided transvaginal reduction. *Ultrasound Obstet. Gynecol.*, **1**, 127–31

77. Venezia, R., Zangara, C., Comparetto, G. and Cittadini, E. (1991). Conservative treatment of ectopic pregnancies using a single echo-guided injection of methotrexate into a gestational sac. *Ultrasound Obstet. Gynecol.*, **1**, 132–5

78. Jehng, C.H., Ng, K.Y., Jou, H.J., Jenh, A.L. and Lien, Y.R. (1992). Successful treatment of two viable tubal pregnancies by two-step local injection. *J. Formos. Med. Assoc.*, **91**, 823–7

79. Atri, M., Bret, P.M., Tulandi, T. and Senterman, M.K. (1992). Ectopic pregnancy: evolution after treatment with transvaginal methotrexate. *Radiology* **185**, 749–53

80. Bider, D., Oelsner, G., Admon, D. *et al.* (1992). Unsuccessful methotrexate treatment of a tubal pregnancy with a live embryo. *Eur. J. Obstet. Gynecol. Reprod. Med.*, **46**, 154–7

81. Caspi, B., Barash, A., Friedman, A., Appelman, Z., Pausky, M. and Borenstein, R. (1992). Aspiration of ectopic pregnancy under guidance of vaginal ultrasonography. *Eur. J. Obstet. Gynecol. Reprod. Biol.*, **46**, 51–2

82. Timor-Tritsch, I.E., Peisner, D.B., Monteagudo, A., Lerner, J.P. and Sharma, S. (1993). Multifetal pregnancy reduction by transvaginal puncture: evaluation of the technique used in 134 cases. *Am. J. Obstet. Gynecol.*, **168**, 799–804

Conservative management of ectopic pregnancy based on color Doppler studies

5

F. Bonilla-Musoles, F. Raga and N. G. Osborne

INTRODUCTION

Up to the 1970s, the diagnosis of ectopic pregnancy was frequently made in women who were hemodynamically unstable due to hemoperitoneum that resulted from tubal rupture. The improvement in sensitivity of methods for detection of the β-subunit of human chorionic gonadotropin (β-hCG) and the development and widespread availability of high-resolution transvaginal ultrasonography made possible earlier diagnosis and, therefore, the conservative management of unruptured Fallopian tubes affected by ectopic pregnancies.

The addition of transvaginal color Doppler sonography promises to refine even more our ability to conserve functional Fallopian tubes, by making it possible for physicians to establish very early on whether a tubal pregnancy is evolutive or regressive. Transvaginal color Doppler is undoubtedly the most comprehensive and sophisticated form of two-dimensional, diagnostic, ultrasonic imaging currently available to health-care professionals for the evaluation of the structure and function of female pelvic structures. The diagnostic information that is gained when transvaginal color Doppler is combined with high-resolution gray-scale B-mode scanning seems to be an improvement over other available forms of two-dimensional sonography.

Research proved that there are changes in the vascular flow impedance of arteries that feed ovulating ovaries. In addition, uterine artery flow impedance recorded at mid-luteal phase is lower than in the follicular phase of the menstrual cycle. These observations suggest that the blood flow to the uterus and the dominant ovary increases during the luteal phase. This increase in blood flow is almost certainly related to the physiological angiogenesis seen in the ovulating ovary and in the endometrium at this phase of the menstrual cycle.

The increased resolution and diagnostic information possible with more sophisticated color Doppler instruments make it possible to determine whether the angiogenesis that occurs in such phenomena like implantation, placentation, and embryogenesis is physiological or pathological.

This information seems to be useful to determine very early whether an ectopic pregnancy is in a state of evolution or regression. Since this information can be obtained before serum β-hCG levels reach the discriminatory zone, it is possible to intervene medically or surgically prior to the time when severe tubal damage or irreversible tubal destruction is likely to occur.

BACKGROUND

The most important gynecological diagnosis to consider in women with an acute abdomen is ectopic pregnancy. Almost 12% of all laparoscopies or laparotomies are performed either to rule out or to treat ectopic pregnancy. Almost one-quarter of urgent gynecological surgical procedures are performed for ectopic pregnancies. Even with techniques currently available, ectopic pregnancy remains a potentially catastrophic complication that results in death for one of every 2000 women affected[1].

The incidence of ectopic pregnancy varies between 0.5 and 1% of all pregnancies. Ten percent of patients with previous tubal pregnancies who still have Fallopian tubes have another ectopic pregnancy[2]. The incidence of ectopic pregnancy continues to increase, mostly due to an increase in the use of assisted reproductive technology. An increase in incidence is also due in part to a higher incidence of sexually acquired diseases. However, due to the emergence of reliable diagnostic methods, such as tranvaginal sonography, and sensitive methods for detection of β-hCG, the mortality associated with ectopic pregnancy has decreased from 3.5/1000 in 1970 to 0.5/1000 in 1980[1]. Newer techniques such as transvaginal color Doppler sonography have the potential to reduce this mortality rate even further.

In the recent past, conservative management of ectopic pregnancy has gained many advocates[2–11]. There are two main reasons for conserving tubes when managing ectopic pregnancies. It is now well established that medical and surgical conservational approaches decrease morbidity and cost[5]. In addition, a high percentage of women with ectopic pregnancy are infertile. It has been shown that many of these women have a reasonable chance of achieving a subsequent intrauterine pregnancy if their Fallopian tubes are conserved[12].

In most published reports about ectopic pregnancies, the diagnosis is established by studying the characteristics of trophoblastic activity by evaluating serial quantitative β-hCG serum levels in patients with a positive pregnancy test in whom an intrauterine gestational sac, with or without recognizable embryonic structures, cannot be seen by ultrasound examination. This is especially true if the initial β-hCG serum levels are below the *discriminatory zone*, i.e. the level of β-hCG at which an intrauterine gestational sac must be seen with ultrasound. This level is 1500–2000 mIU/ml, or approximately 5 weeks of amenorrhea (about 2–4 mm embryonic size) using transvaginal sonography.

Once a diagnosis of ectopic pregnancy is made, the physician has to decide on an appropriate plan of management. There are several reports about spontaneous resolution of ectopic pregnancies[13–16]. In selected cases, spontaneous resolution ranges between 64 and 92%[17,18]. These figures suggest that, under very specific conditions, certain patients with a diagnosis of ectopic pregnancy can be managed with expectant observation[13].

We recognize that the diagnostic algorithms and methods suggested for the management of ectopic pregnancy by expectant observation are not yet clearly established. However, recent data suggest that, depending on the clinical situation, selected patients with an ectopic pregnancy may be observed by monitoring the evolution of symptoms, by following serial biochemical determinations of β-hCG, and by monitoring adnexal mass size and vascular flow changes with serial transvaginal ultrasonic and color Doppler flow scans[6,10,13,19–46]. An increase in β-hCG levels has been related to actively growing or *progressing* ectopic pregnancy. When β-hCG levels plateau or actually decrease, the evidence is that the ectopic pregnancy is *regressing*[17,18]. Likewise, a decrease in resistance index (RI) or in pulsatility index (PI) is evidence of a developing ectopic pregnancy, while an increase in RI and PI has been associated with a regressive ectopic pregnancy[13].

In managing patients by expectant observation, it is necessary to recognize that the correlation between β-hCG levels and the actual *vitality* of trophoblast tissue in an ectopic pregnancy is not always linear. There are reports of tubal pregnancies which have ruptured in the presence of decreasing or 'non-pregnant' plasma levels of β-hCG[16,47–52].

As Doppler ultrasound analyzes trophoblast and flow to the corpus luteum[21,24,25,28,29,35,42,45,46,53,54], several investigators have recognized the possibility of monitoring ectopic pregnancies with transvaginal color Doppler sonography when expectant observation was considered appropriate. Moreover, since color Doppler velocity waveforms correspond with corpus luteum production of estradiol and progesterone[7,55–57], a fundamental process for the maintenance of gestation in the early stages, corpus luteum flow measurement could also be a good parameter for establishing the developing or regressive nature of an ectopic pregnancy[46]. Preliminary results suggest that it is possible to identify reliably living and regressing ectopic pregnancies by monitoring trophoblastic and corpus luteum activity with transvaginal color Doppler sonography. In fact, the evidence is that transvaginal color Doppler is more sensitive than serial plasma β-hCG for the correct identification of developing and regressive ectopic pregnancies[13–15, 19, 44, 47, 58–74] (Color plates 4 and 5).

By combining transvaginal sonography with color Doppler, it is possible to detect the presence or absence of cul-de-sac fluid and the presence or absence of 'flow imaging' in the adnexal mass and in the corpus luteum. If the characteristic vascular flow of neoangiogenesis associated with trophoblastic tissue is detected in the adnexal mass, this is objective evidence of an ectopic pregnancy. The RI and PI of the adnexal mass, of the corpus luteum, and of the uterine arteries are then monitored to determine whether the ectopic pregnancy shows evidence of development or of regression. Current data indicate that adnexal mass and corpus luteum RI values > 0.45 and PI values > 0.75 are the discriminatory cut-off values between developing and regressive ectopic pregnancies. Histological examination of trophoblastic tissue has demonstrated that flow indices below these may correlate at times with active trophoblastic tissue, while greater flow indices may correlate with degenerated villi[74]. According to these recent data, it is therefore possible to identify ectopic pregnancies in regression that do not require surgical intervention[13, 57, 75].

Clearly, surgical or medical intervention is necessary when monitoring by expectant observation is not an option. If surgical intervention is indicated, the question is then whether a laparoscopic approach is an option or whether a laparotomy is necessary.

ULTRASOUND DIAGNOSIS OF ECTOPIC PREGNANCY

Transvaginal sonography findings

A review of the world literature indicates that transvaginal sonography has a diagnostic sensitivity between 75 and 90% for the diagnosis of ectopic pregnancy. The following images may be seen:

(1) An empty uterus (27.8%);

(2) An empty uterus and an adnexal mass (34.7%);

(3) An intrauterine sac or pseudogestational sac (25%);

(4) An empty uterus and an ectopic gestational sac (12.5%) with or without:

    (a) A yolk sac,

    (b) An embryo,

    (c) Embryonic heart activity;

(5) Images (1)–(4) with cul-de-sac 'fluid' (25%).

The sonographic image observed will depend both on gestational age and on whether the ectopic pregnancy is in development or in regression at the time when it is first diagnosed. The evidence is that at least 60% of ectopic pregnancies regress spontaneously. Regressive ectopic pregnancies only present the images described in (1) and (2). Only rarely is the image described in (3) seen with regressive ectopic pregnancies. Therefore, in cases of early diagnosis, living embryos are observed infrequently. This observation is so well established that it can be stated with confidence that, if a living embryo is seen in a Fallopian tube, the diagnosis may have been made late.

The images described in (3) and (4) have a diagnostic sensitivity of 100%. With amenorrhea for more than 35 days and β-hCG values greater than 650 mIU/ml, the images described in (1) and (2) have a diagnostic sensitivity of 80%. In cases where ectopic pregnancy is suspected by the observation of images (1) and (2), the diagnosis can be confirmed or ruled out by clinical and sonographic re-evaluations every 3 or 4 days. This monitoring can be done in an ambulatory setting when patients are adequately counselled and informed.

Transvaginal color Doppler sonography is of little diagnostic value when an intrauterine pseudogestational sac or an ectopic gestational sac is recognized. The diagnostic sensitivity and specificity of ultrasound are excellent in these cases. Since the diagnosis is established when a pseudogestational sac is identified by sonography, transvaginal color Doppler sonography is only useful to establish whether the ectopic pregnancy is in development or in regression. Transvaginal color Doppler sonography is useless when there is sonographic identification of an ectopic yolk sac or detection of an embryo or of cardiac activity. In these cases, the developing nature of the ectopic pregnancy is obvious and immediate therapeutic intervention is necessary.

Detection of an 'empty uterus' in a patient with detectable levels of β-hCG is usually associated with a uterus with decidual endometrium. In other words, there is a thick, homogeneous, and well demarcated endometrial line without a gestational sac[25]. In patients with positive levels of β-hCG, this transvaginal ultrasound image of the endometrium has a diagnostic sensitivity of 80% for ectopic pregnancy. It is one of the most important sonographic findings suggestive of ectopic pregnancy.

It is important to remember that the so-called intrauterine 'pseudogestational sac' results from a low sonographic resolution power, from the homogeneous ultrasonic impedance of decidua, and from fluid collection in the center of the intrauterine decidual layer. This image, and therefore the use of this term, is restricted only to transabdominal sonography.

The presence of fluid in the cul-de-sac is a finding that helps to establish the diagnosis of ectopic pregnancy. However, this finding is only of limited value, since it appears in only 25% of ectopic pregnancies. Furthermore, experienced laparoscopists are aware that many women, including women who are anovulatory or menopausal, may have fluid collection in the pouch of Douglas which originates from omental transudate.

False-positive and false-negative findings

Certain factors may contribute to false-positive or false-negative results with transvaginal ultrasonography[16]. The following merit consideration:

(1) The most common reason for false-positive findings is due to erroneous information about the period of amenorrhea or due to a lack of knowledge about the menstrual formula (Kaltenbach's menogram). However, this problem can be solved easily with successive analytical and sonographic controls;

(2) The presence of hemoperitoneum can interfere with the sonographic field of vision;

(3) Heterotopic gestations;

(4) Double ectopic gestations;

(5) Early spontaneous abortion with low levels of residual β-hCG.

Transvaginal color Doppler findings

Except for a few authors[19,43], most investigators agree that the addition of transvaginal color Doppler sonography improves the diagnostic sensitivity for the detection of ectopic pregnancy[6,10,20-46]. In our experience, the diagnostic sensitivity of ultrasound for the early detection of ectopic pregnancy increases from 80 to 90% with the addition of transvaginal color Doppler sonography. The reason for this improvement is that, in addition to detection of the adnexal mass, transvaginal color Doppler sonography evalutes the following:

(1) The appearance of trophoblastic 'flow imaging';

(2) The RI and PI of trophoblastic flow velocity curves;

(3) Corpus luteum flow indices.

Normal values

The velocity curves of ectopic pregnancy flow have characteristic high diastolic levels. These levels are identical to the trophoblastic flows observed when there is an intrauterine pregnancy. They are also similar to the flows observed in the gestational corpus luteum. For this reason, it is important to observe *separately* the flows of the ectopic trophoblastic tissue and of the corpus luteum in order to avoid false-positive conclusions. In our experience, over 90% of ectopic pregnancies implant in the Fallopian tube on the side of the ovary that has the gestational corpus luteum. This fact is likely to facilitate diagnostic errors.

Due to the great vascular activity that is taking place, the type of flow that is seen in an ectopic pregnancy, even when observed in the early stages, is very irregular and colorful (Color plates 4 and 5). Although the flow in the corpus luteum can also be very colorful, the trophoblastic flow is different from the flow observed in the corpus luteum in the sense that the corpus luteum has a flow that is circular or semi-circular, the so-called 'half moon' pattern (Color plates 6 and 7). The reason for the semi-circular flow pattern is that it results from newly formed vessels in the luteinized theca granulosa layer. The identification of these patterns should therefore raise the suspicion that one is observing corpus luteum flow and not trophoblastic flow.

The flow values observed in trophoblastic flow are always equal to or less than 0.45 for the resistance index and equal to or less than 0.75 for the pulsatility index. These values are similar to those found in the gestational corpus luteum.

In our experience, flow imaging is observed in 88% of ectopic pregnancies with an 'empty uterus' or with an adnexal mass. In the case of an 'empty uterus', the presence of adnexal flow imaging with transvaginal color Doppler sonography establishes the diagnosis of ectopic pregnancy. With transvaginal ultrasound alone, an 'empty uterus' by itself is always a 'false-negative' finding that leads to a suspicion of ectopic pregnancy.

In a few cases where there is an ectopic pregnancy, flow imaging may not be seen with transvaginal color Doppler sonography if any of the following conditions is present:

(1) Very early gestational age;

(2) Presence of a regressing ectopic pregnancy;

(3) Presence of significant hemoperitoneum.

Corpus luteum flow imaging, observed in 76% of early ectopic pregnancies, is especially important for the determination of evolution or regression in an ectopic pregnancy. The reasons for not observing corpus luteum flow imaging are:

(1) False-negative (exceptionally rare);

(2) Regressive corpus luteum;

(3) Ovaries beyond the sonographic visual field;

(4) Significant hemoperitoneum.

False-positive and false-negative findings

Special care must be taken to avoid the following reasons for false-positive and false-negative results:

(1) Confusion of a corpus luteum with an ectopic pregnancy;

(2) The presence of multiple corpora lutea. It must be kept in mind that 25% of the ectopic pregnancies we identified occurred in patients who underwent one of the regimens of assisted reproduction that involved ovulation induction. In cases of ovulation induction, multiple corpora lutea are normal;

(3) The presence of a corpus luteum and an incidental cyst;

(4) The presence of an ectopic pregnancy and a hydrosalpinx;

(5) Unconfirmed biochemical pregnancies (as in *in vitro* fertilization and embryo transfer);

(6) Postabortal syncytial endometritis;

(7) Tubal decidualization;

Table 1 Transvaginal sonography: effect of color Doppler on diagnostic sensitivity

Gestational age (weeks)	Number of cases	Transvaginal sonography			Transvaginal color Doppler sonography			
		Positive	*Negative*	*% positive*	*Positive*	*Negative*	*% positive*	*p*
4	7	3	4	42.8	4	3	57.1	1.00
5	17	12	5	70.6	13	4	76.5	0.71
6	24	18	6	75.0	21	3	87.5	0.45
7	19	15	4	78.9	17	2	89.5	0.65
8	5	4	1	80.0	4	1	80.0	0.41
Total	72	52	20	72.2	59	13	81.9	0.54

Table 2 Diagnostic accuracy of transvaginal sonography and transvaginal color Doppler sonography for gestational ages more and less than 7 weeks

Gestational age (weeks)	Number of cases	Transvaginal sonography			Transvaginal color Doppler sonography			
		Positive	Negative	% positive	Positive	Negative	% positive	p
<7	48	33	15	68.8	38	10	79.2	0.48
>7	24	19	5	79.2	21	3	87.5	1.0

Table 3 Corpus luteum vascular flow imaging: accuracy of transvaginal color Doppler sonography by gestational age

Gestational age (weeks)	Number of cases	Corpus luteum flow imaging		
		Positive	Negative	% positive
4	7	7	0	100
5	17	13	4	76.4
6	24	21	3	87.9
7	19	12	7	63.1
8	5	4	1	80.0
Total	72	57	15	79.1

(8) Bilateral ectopic pregnancy;

(9) Heterotopic pregnancy;

(10) Lack of knowledge about the period of amenorrhea or of Kaltenbach's menogram.

RI and PI values in the area of ectopic implantation

In our experience, flow imaging in the area of implantation can be observed in 80% of ectopic pregnancies investigated. The ability to observe flow imaging is dependent on gestational age (Table 1). The RI and PI values that have been observed are: RI, 0.44 ± 0.10 (range 0.25–0.83); PI, 0.70 ± 0.22 (range 0.32–1.53). Although there is a tendency for RI and PI values to decrease as the age of ectopic pregnancies increases, the differences are not statistically significant. The only significance of decreasing or increasing values in serial determinations is the identification of developing or regressive ectopic pregnancies.

Combination of transvaginal sonography and color Doppler sonography

The diagnostic sensitivity with the exclusive use of transvaginal sonography is 72.2% and that of transvaginal color Doppler sonography exclusively is 81.9%. The difference is not statistically significant. However, there is a reduction in the false-positive and false-negative results inherent with each modality when these techniques are used to complement each other so that, when combined, the diagnostic sensitivity varies between 88 and 95%.

Diagnostic accuracy related to gestational age

We have mentioned that the sonographic image evolves with the temporal development of an ectopic pregnancy. For this reason, when early diagnoses are made, certain images like an adnexal mass are seen more frequently than

Table 4 Relationship between gestational age of ectopic pregnancy and β-hCG serum levels (mIU/ml)

Gestational age (weeks)	Number of cases	Mean	Minimum	Maximum	Standard deviation
4	7	936.4	48	2187	± 985
5	17	1176.5	187	6727	± 1602
6	24	1494.3	94	14324	± 2896
7	19	2387.3	48	6330	± 2130
8	5	3751.2	106	7900	± 3767
Total	72	1784	48	14324	± 2443

Table 5 'Developing' and 'regressive' ectopic pregnancies: differences in β-hCG levels. The numbers of ectopic pregnancies are in parentheses

Gestational age (weeks)	Mean β-hCG level (mIU/ml)		p
	Developing	Regressive	
4	936 (5)	53 (2)	0.02*
5	1719 (8)	639 (9)	0.2
6	2582 (11)	496 (13)	0.08
7	3528 (12)	819 (7)	0.003*
8	6150 (3)	154 (2)	0.05*

* Statistically significant difference

other images like the embryo. As the experience of sonographers improves, earlier diagnoses based on images that do not rely on direct visualization of the embryo can be expected. Likewise, observation and evaluation of adnexal mass flow velocity curves are dependent on gestational age and β-hCG levels. The diagnostic accuracy of transvaginal sonography improves with the age of an ectopic pregnancy (Tables 2 and 3).

As is the case with transvaginal sonography, diagnostic accuracy increases with transvaginal color Doppler sonography with the age of an ectopic pregnancy. Although differences are not statistically significant, diagnostic accuracy improves when the gestational age is greater than 7 weeks (Table 2).

β-hCG values

During the past year, we have examined the quantitative β-hCG levels of 72 women with ectopic pregnancies. The average level was 1784 mIU/ml with a range of 48–14 324 mIU/ml. Although the data in Tables 4 and 5 are averages, it was of interest that 45 of the 72 women with ectopic pregnancies had β-hCG levels below 1500 mIU/ml and 37 had levels below 1000 mIU/ml, although only 24 women had pregnancies of 5 weeks or less since their last menstrual period.

If we compare levels of β-hCG between developing and regressive ectopic pregnancies as a group, the differences are statistically significant (Table 5). Analyzed by weeks of amenorrhea, the differences approach statistical significance for women at weeks 5 and 6 of amenorrhea and are statistically significant for women at weeks 4, 7 and 8 of amenorrhea.

Regardless of the developing or regressive nature of ectopic pregnancies, β-hCG levels do not follow the classicial increasing pattern seen with intrauterine pregnancies. The β-hCG levels do not double in the predictable way that they double with intrauterine pregnancies. These observations are in agreement with recent reports that suggest that high levels of β-hCG are not frequently seen with ectopic pregnancies[14,15].

In our series, the mean level of serum β-hCG on days 30–38 after the last menstrual period was 1056.45 mIU/ml (range 48–1916). The mean level of β-hCG before the appearance of adnexal mass vascular flow was 263.5 mIU/ml (range 51–619). The mean before disappearance of the vascular image in regressive ectopics was 233.8 mIU/ml with a range of 48–600 mIU/ml. In other words, in all cases studied where there were 34 days of amenorrhea and the β-hCG serum levels were equal to, or exceeded 600 mIU/ml, there was vascular imaging in the adnexal mass. These data are important, since they reduce the diagnostic 'cut off' to 35 days of amenorrhea even with β-hCG serum levels of 600 mIU/ml, which is well below the old 'discriminatory zone' for detection of an endometrial gestational sac.

Our data indicate that, with ectopic pregnancies, there is a definite relationship between serum β-hCG levels and the appearance of adnexal flow imaging. At β-hCG serum levels below those at which adnexal mass flow imaging is visible, there is no statistically significant difference between the β-hCG serum levels of patients with developing and those with regressive ectopic pregnancies. Since β-hCG serum levels are not reliable indicators of an ectopic pregnancy below the 'discriminatory zone', observation and evaluation of the flow characteristics of the adnexal mass, even with β-hCG serum levels between 600 mIU/ml and 1500 mIU/ml, are more useful to establish if an ectopic pregnancy is in development or in regression.

CONCLUSIONS

The current 'gold standard' for conservative management of ectopic pregnancy depends on the early identification of the ectopic gestation by quantitative β-hCG assays, serum progesterone assays, and on transvaginal sonography when β-hCG assays are above the 'discriminatory zone'. Conservative surgical management, usually through a laparoscopic approach, is considered appropriate for patients desirous of future pregnancy who have an intact gestational sac in the Fallopian tube or who have sufficient salvageable Fallopian tube even in the case of rupture. Women with unruptured ectopic pregnancies of less than 3 cm and without evidence of fetal cardiac activity may be treated with methotrexate, a folic acid inhibitor that blocks nucleic acid synthesis in the trophoblast.

With the addition of transvaginal color Doppler sonography to the diagnostic armamentarium of gynecologists, it is now possible to make an early diagnosis of regressive ectopic pregnancy by identification of adnexal mass and corpus luteum flows with increasing resistance and pulsatility indices. Our data suggest that, for purposes of management, systematic evaluation of the flow indices of the corpus luteum and of the adnexal mass provides more important indicators of a developing ectopic pregnancy or one in regression, than does serial quantitative serum β-hCG assay.

References

1. Rubin, G.L., Peterson, H.B., Porfman, S.F., Layde, P.M., Ware, J.M., Ory, H.W. and Cartes, W. (1983). Ectopic pregnancy in the United States: 1970 through 1978. *J. Am. Med. Assoc.*, **249**, 1725–8

2. Simon, C., Sampaio, M., Pardo, G., Matallin, P. and Bonilla-Musoles, F. (1989). Tratamiento conservador del embarazo ectópico. Revisión de conjunto. *Rev. Españ. Obstet. Ginecol.*, **48**, 43–50

3. Atri, M., Bret, P.M., Tulandi, T. and Senterman, M.K. (1992). Ectopic pregnancy: evolution after treatment with transvaginal methotrexate. *Radiology*, **185**, 749–53

4. Brown, D.L., Felker, R.E., Stovall, T.G., Emerson, D.S. and Ling, F.N. (1991). Serial endovaginal sonography of ectopic pregnancies treated with methotrexate. *Obstet. Gynecol.*, **77**, 406–9

5. Brumsted, J., Kessler, C., Gibson, C., Nakajima, S., Riddick, D.H. and Gibson, M.A. (1988). Comparison of laparoscopy and laparotomy for the treatment of ectopic pregnancy. *Obstet. Gynecol.*, **71**, 889–92

6. Kirchler, A., Alge, A., Huter, O. and Schwegel, P. (1992). Blood flow measurement in ectopic pregnancy before and after prostaglandin injection: a therapy control. *Ultrasound Obstet. Gynecol.*, **2** (Suppl.), 118

7. Kuhlman, K.A., Arnaud, S., Ninkel, C.A. and Sobel, M.I. (1992). Longitudinal transvaginal ultrasound studies of ectopic pregnancies in women receiving outpatient methotrexate therapy. *J. Ultrasound Med.*, **11**, 40s

8. Lundorff, P., Hahlin, M., Sjoblon, P. and Lindblon, B. (1991). Persistent trophoblast after conservative treatment of tubal pregnancy: prediction and detection. *Obstet. Gynecol.*, **77**, 129–33

9. Thompson, G.R., O'Shea, R.T. and Seman, E. (1991). Methotrexate injection of tubal ectopic pregnancy: a logical evolution? *Med. J. Aust.*, **154**, 469–71

10. Tekay, A. and Jouppila, P. (1992). Color Doppler flow as an indicator of trophoblastic activity in tubal pregnancies detected by transvaginal ultrasound. *Obstet. Gynecol.*, **80**, 995–9

11. Ylöstalo, P., Cacciatore, B., Sjöberg, J., Kääriäinen, M., Tenhunen, A. and Stenman, U.H. (1992). Expectant management of ectopic pregnancy. *Obstet. Gynecol.*, **80**, 345–8

12. Stovall, T.G., Ling, F.W., Gray, L.A., Carson, S.A. and Burter, J.E. (1991). Methotrexate treatment of unruptured ectopic pregnancy: a report of 100 cases. *Obstet. Gynecol.*, **77**, 749–53

13. Bonilla-Musoles, F., Ballester, M.J., Tarin, J.J., Raga, F., Osborne, N.G. and Pellicer, A. (1995). Does transvaginal color Doppler sonography differentiate between developing and involuting ectopic pregnancy? *J. Ultrasound Med.*, **14**, 175–82

14. Cacciatore, B., Stenman, U.H. and Ylöstalo, P. (1990). Diagnosis of ectopic pregnancy by transvaginal ultrasonography in combination with discriminatory serum β-hCG level of 1000 IU/l (IRP). *Br. J. Obstet. Gynaecol.*, **97**, 904–8

15. Cacciatore, B. (1991). Early diagnosis of ectopic pregnancy by ultrasonography and quantitative determination of serum hCG. *Acta Obstet. Gynecol. Scand.*, **70**, 633–4

16. Parvey, R. and Maklad, N. (1993). Pitfalls in the transvaginal sonographic diagnosis of ectopic pregnancy. *J. Ultrasound Med.*, **12**, 139–44

17. Fernandez, H., Rainhorn, J.B., Papernik, E., Bellet, D. and Frydman, R. (1988). Spontaneous resolution of ectopic pregnancy. *Obstet. Gynecol.*, **71**, 171–4

18. Garcia, A.J., Aubert, J.M., Sama, J. and Josimovich, J.B. (1987). Expectant management of presumed ectopic pregnancies. *Fertil. Steril.*, **48**, 395–400

19. Achiron, R., Goldenberg, M., Oelsner, G., Lipitz, S. and Mashiach, S. (1992). Transvaginal duplex Doppler ultrasonography in evaluating ectopic pregnancy. *Ultrasound Obstet. Gynecol.*, **2** (Suppl.), 62

20. Atkinson, P. and Wells, P. (1977). Pulse-Doppler ultrasound and its clinical application. *Yale J. Biol. Med.*, **50**, 367–73

21. Alfirevic, Z. and Kurjak, A. (1990). Transvaginal color and pulsed wave Doppler in the assessment of blood flow in the first trimester of pregnancy. *J. Perinatol. Med.*, **18**, 173–9

22. Asseryanis, E., Schurz, B., Eppel, W., Frigo, P., Adler, A., Husslein, P. and Reinold, E. (1993). Spätkomplikation einer Tuybargravidität dargestellt mit der Farb-Doppler Sonographie. Eine Kasuistik. *Ultraschall*, **14**, 180–1

23. Bourne, T.H. (1991). Transvaginal color Doppler in gynecology. *Ultrasound Obstet. Gynecol.*, **1**, 359–73

24. Bourne, T.H., Jurkovic, D., Reynolds, K., Campbell, S. and Collins, W.P. (1992). A comparison of the changes in pelvic blood flow in early uterine pregnancies and ectopic pregnancies. *J. Ultrasound Med.*, **11**, 41s

25. Bonilla-Musoles, F., Ballester, M.J. and Carreras, J.M. (1992). *Doppler Color Transvaginal*, pp. 59–63, (Barcelona: Masson-Salvat)

26. Bonilla-Musoles, F. and Ballester, M.J. (1992). Transvaginal color Doppler in the diagnosis of ectopic pregnancy. *Ultrasound Obstet. Gynecol.*, **2** (Suppl.), 72

27. Csabay, L., Szabó, I., Német, J., Sipos, Z.S. and Papp, Z. (1992). The use of color Doppler transvaginal ultrasound in the monitoring of ectopic pregnancy. *Ultrasound Obstet. Gynecol.*, **2** (Suppl.), 82

28. Dillon, E.H. and Taylor, K.J. (1990). Doppler ultrasound in the female pelvis and first trimester of pregnancy. *Clin. Diagn. Ultrasound*, **26**, 93–117

29. Dillon, E.H., Feycock, A.L. and Taylor, K.J. (1990). Pseudogestational sacs: Doppler US differentiation from normal or abnormal intrauterine pregnancies. *Radiology*, **176**, 359–64

30. Emerson, D.S., Cartier, M.S., Altieri, L.A., Felker, R.E., Smith, W.C.H., Stovall, T.G. and Gray, L.A. (1992). Diagnostic efficacy of endovaginal color Doppler flow imaging in an ectopic pregnancy screening program. *Radiology*, **183**, 413–20

31. Jurkovic, D., Bourne, T.H., Jauniaux, E., Campbell, S. and Collins, W.P. (1992). Transvaginal color Doppler study of blood flow in ectopic pregnancies. *Fertil. Steril.*, **57**, 68–73

32. Kirchler, H.C.L., Kölle, D. and Schwegel, P. (1992). Changes in tubal blood flow in evaluating ectopic pregnancy. *Ultrasound Obstet. Gynecol.*, **2**, 283–8

33. Kurjak, A. and Zalud, I. (1990). Transvaginaler Farbdoppler für die Beurteilung von gynäkologischen Pathologien in kleinen Becken. *Ultraschall. Med.*, **11**, 164–8

34. Kurjak, A., Zalud, I., Alfirevic, Z. and Jurkovic, D. (1990). The assessment of abnormal pelvic blood flow by transvaginal color and pulsed Doppler. *Ultrasound Med. Biol.*, **16**, 437–42

35. Kurjak, A. (1990). *Transvaginal Color Doppler*. (Carnforth, UK: Parthenon)

36. Kurjak, A., Jurkovic, D., Alfirevic, Z. and Zalud, I. (1990). Transvaginal color Doppler imaging. *J. Clin. Ultrasound*, **18**, 227–34

37. Kurjak, A., Zalud, I. and Schulman, H. (1991). Ectopic pregnancy: transvaginal color Doppler of trophoblastic flow in questionable adnexa. *J. Ultrasound Med.*, **10**, 685–9

38. Kurjak, A. and Zalud, I. (1992). Ultrasound assessment of ectopic pregnancy. In Jaffe, R. and Warsof, S.L. (eds.) *Color Doppler Imaging in Obstetrics and Gynecology*, pp. 85–98. (New York: McGraw-Hill)

39. Pellerito, J.S., Taylor, K.J., Quedens-Case, C., Hammers, L.W., Scoutt, L.M., Ramos, I.M. and Meyer, W.R. (1992). Ectopic pregnancy: evaluation with endovaginal color flow imaging. *Radiology*, **183**, 407–11

40. Schurz, B., Wenzl, R., Eppel, W., Asseryanis, E. and Reinold, E. (1993). Blutflussemssungen von Neovaskularisationen bei Tubargravidität. *Ultraschall*, **14**, 178–9

41. Stabile, I., Grudzinskas, J. and Campbell, S. (1990). Doppler ultrasonographic evaluation of abnormal pregnancies in the first trimester. *J. Clin. Ultrasound*, **18**, 497–501

42. Stabile, I., Grudzinskas, J. and Campbell, S. (1990). Pulsed Doppler as applied to maternal circulation in normal and failed first trimester pregnancy. *Echocardiography*, **6**, 353–6

43. Stella-Troche, V., Quere, M.P., Laurent, F.X., Laborde, O., Mensier, A. and Lopes, P. (1993). Interet du Doppler couleur dans les diagnostics difficiles de grossesse extra-uterine. *J. Gynecol. Obstet. Biol. Reprod.*, **22**, 896–7

44. Taylor, K.J.W., Ramos, I.M., Fayock, A.L., Snower, D.P., Carter, D., Shapiro, B.S., Meyer, W.R. and DeCherney, A.H. (1989). Ectopic pregnancy: duplex Doppler evaluation. *Radiology*, **173**, 93–9

45. Thaler, I., Manor, D., Itskovitz, J., Rottem, S., Levitt, N., Timor-Tritsch, I. and Bandres, I.M. (1990). Changes in uterine blood flow during human pregnancy. *Am. J. Obstet. Gynecol.*, **162**, 121–5

46. Zalud, I. and Kurjak, A. (1990). The assessment of luteal blood flow in pregnant and non pregnant women by transvaginal color Doppler. *J. Perinatol.*, **18**, 215–20

47. Ankum, W.M., Van Der Veen, F., Hamerlynck, J.V.T. and Lammes, F.B. (1993). Transvaginal sonography and human chorionic gonadotrophin measurements in suspected ectopic pregnancy: a detailed analysis of a diagnostic approach. *Hum. Reprod.*, **8**, 1307–11

48. Hochner-Celnikier, D., Ron, M., Goshen, R., Zacut, D., Mair, G. and Yagel, S. (1992). Rupture of ectopic pregnancy following disappearance of serum beta subunit of hCG. *Obstet. Gynecol.*, **79**, 826–7

49. Moccato, M., Estrada, R. and Faro, S. (1993). Ectopic pregnancy with undetectable serum and urine β-hCG levels and detection of β-hCG in the ectopic trophoblast by immunocytochemical evaluation. *Obstet. Gynecol.*, **81**, 878–80

50. Schiff, E., Ben-Baruch, G., Moran, O., Yahal, I., Oelsner, G., Mashiach, S. and Menczer, J. (1990). Prediction of residual trophoblastic tissue in first trimester abortion and low levels of human chorionic gonadotropin β-subunit. *Am. J. Obstet. Gynecol.*, **162**, 797–801

51. Taylor, R., Padula, C. and Goldsmith, P. (1988). Pitfall in the diagnosis of ectopic pregnancy: immunocytochemical evaluation in a patient with false-negative serum β-hCG levels. *Obstet. Gynecol.*, **71**, 1035–8

52. Tulandi, T., Hemmings, R. and Khalifa, F. (1991). Rupture of ectopic pregnancy in women with low and declining serum β-human chorionic gonadotropin concentrations. *Fertil. Steril.*, **56**, 786–7

53. Januiaux, E., Jurkovic, D. and Campbell, S. (1991). *In vivo* investigation of the anatomy and the physiology of early human placental circulations. *Ultrasound Obstet. Gynecol.*, **1**, 435–45

54. Schaaps, J.P., Mustin, J. and Lambotte, R. (1991). Vaginosonographische Aspekte der Uterus Trophoblastzirkulation. In Popp, L.W. (ed.) *Gynäkologische Endosonographie*, pp. 127–32. (Quickborn: Klemke Verlag).

55. Bustillo, M., Stern, J.J., King, D. and Coulam, C.B. (1993). Serum progesterone and estradiol concentrations in the early diagnosis of ectopic pregnancy after *in vitro* fertilization–embryo transfer. *Fertil. Steril.*, **59**, 668–70

56. Csapó, A.I., Pulkinen, K.O. and Wiest, W.G. (1993). Effects of luteectomy and progesterone replacement therapy in early pregnant patients. *Am. J. Obstet. Gynecol.*, **115**, 759–64

57. Guillaume, J., Benjamin, F., Sicuranza, B., Wang, C.F., Garcia, A. and Friberg, J. (1987). Maternal serum levels of estradiol, progesterone and human chorionic gonadotropin in ectopic pregnancy and their correlation with endometrial histologic findings. *Surg. Gynecol. Obstet.*, **165**, 9–12

58. Bonilla-Musoles, F. (1992). *Tratado de endosonografía en obstetricia y ginecología*, pp. 134–56. (Barcelona: Masson-Salvat)

59. Brown, D.L. and Doubilet, P.M. (1994). Transvaginal sonography for diagnosing ectopic pregnancy: positivity criteria and performance characteristic. *J. Ultrasound Med.*, **13**, 259–66

60. Enk, L., Wikland, M., Hammerberg, K. and Lindblom, B. (1990). The value of endovaginal sonography and urinary human chorionic gonadotropin test for differentiation between intrauterine and ectopic pregnancy. *J. Clin. Ultrasound*, **18**, 73–8

61. Filly, R.A. (1987). Ectopic pregnancy: the role of sonography. *Radiology*, **162**, 661–8

62. Gabrielli, S. and Romero, R. (1992). Accuracy of transvaginal ultrasound and serum hCG in the diagnosis of ectopic pregnancy. *Ultrasound Obstet. Gynecol.*, **2**, 110–15

63. Kadar, N., DeVore, G. and Romero, R. (1981). Discriminatory hCG zone: its use in the sono-

graphic evaluation for ectopic pregnancy. *Obstet. Gynecol.*, **58**, 156–61

64. Mahony, B.S., Filly, R.A., Nyberg, D.A. and Cullen, P. (1985). Sonographic evaluation of ectopic pregnancy. *J. Ultrasound Med.*, **4**, 221–7

65. Nyberg, D.A., Filly, R.A., Laing, F.C., Mack, I.A. and Zarutskie, P.W. (1987). Ectopic pregnancy: diagnosis by sonography correlated with quantitative hCG levels. *J. Ultrasound Med.*, **6**, 145–50

66. Nyberg, D.A., Mack, J.A., Laing, F.C. *et al.* (1988). Early pregnancy complications: endovaginal sonographic findings correlated with human chorionic gonadotropin levels. *Radiology*, **197**, 619–24

67. Nyberg, D.A., Hughes, M.P., Mack, L.A. and Wang, K.Y. (1991). Extrauterine findings of ectopic pregnancy at transvaginal US: importance of echogenic fluid. *Radiology*, **178**, 823–6

68. Popp, L.W., Colditz, A. and Gaetje, R. (1993). Diagnosis of intrauterine and ectopic pregnancy at 5–7 postmenstrual weeks. *Int. J. Gynecol. Obstet.*, **44**, 33–8

69. Rempen, A. (1988). Vaginal sonography in ectopic pregnancy: a positive evaluation. *J. Ultrasound Med.*, **7**, 381–7

70. Romero, R., Kadar, N., Castro, D., Jeanty, P., Hobbins, J.C. and DeCherney, A. (1988). The value of adnexal sonographic findings in the diagnosis of ectopic pregnancy. *Am. J. Obstet. Gynecol.*, **158**, 52–7

71. Russel, S.A., Filly, R.A. and Damato, N. (1993). Sonographic diagnosis of ectopic pregnancy with endovaginal probes: what really has changed? *J. Ultrasound Med.*, **12**, 145–52

72. Thorsen, M.K., Lawson, T.L., Atman, E.J. *et al.* (1990). Diagnosis of ectopic pregnancy: endovaginal versus transabdominal sonography. *Am. J. Roentgenol.*, **155**, 307–10

73. Wiedemann, R., Strowitzki, T., Sandner, R., Luppa, P. and Hepp, H. (1989). Wertigkeit hormoneller und sonographischer Parameter bei der Diagnostik der gestörten bzw. ungestörten Frühgravidität. *Geburtsh. Frauenheilk.*, **49**, 237–42

74. Salim, A., Zalud, I., Farmakides, G., Schulman, H., Kurjak, A. and Latin, V. (1994). Corpus luteum blood flow in normal and abnormal early pregnancy: evaluation with transvaginal color pulsed Doppler sonography. *J. Ultrasound Med.*, **13**, 971–5

75. Blaustein, A. (1977). *Pathology of the Female Genital Tract*, pp. 646–55. (New York: Springer)

Inflammatory processes of the Fallopian tube

6

J. P. Lerner, I. E. Timor-Tritsch and A. Monteagudo

INTRODUCTION

Although normal Fallopian tubes evade traditional sonographic scrutiny except with the presence of a small amount of pelvic fluid, diseased tubes secondary to infectious processes are easily identified using high-resolution transvaginal sonography. Correct identification of Fallopian tube pathology is achieved by evaluating the structure of the tubal wall, the luminal contents and the relationship of the tube to the surrounding pelvic structures. Most infectious tubal lesions are associated with the presence of increased quantities of pelvic fluid, allowing for better visualization of small tubal structures. The primary sonographic diagnoses seen are pyosalpinx or hydrosalpinx and tubo-ovarian abscess or complex, both secondary to pelvic inflammatory disease (PID).

ETIOLOGY AND PATHOPHYSIOLOGY

Pelvic inflammatory disease is actually a group of inflammatory processes involving the upper genital tract, including infection of any, several, or all of the following locations: endometrium (endometritis) and/or myometrium (myometritis), Fallopian tubes (salpingitis), ovary (oophoritis), the broad ligaments (parametritis), or pelvic peritoneum (peritonitis). Most authors and clinicians prefer using the term PID or salpingitis, because Fallopian tube involvement is the most common and characteristic component. PID is a serious complication of sexually transmitted bacterial infection that can cause permanent damage to the upper reproductive tract, leading to infertility, ectopic pregnancy and chronic pelvic pain.

In the past, the most frequent causative agent of PID was *Neisseria gonorrheae*. However, *Chlamydia trachomatis* is now the most common infectious organism: the Centers for Disease Control estimate that *C. trachomatis* is responsible for one-quarter to one-half of all cases of PID[1]. *Chlamydia* is the organism that is most closely associated with the serious and long-term sequelae of PID.

Pelvic inflammatory disease is the result of an infection, usually by *N. gonorrheae* or *Chlamydia*, ascending from the lower to the upper genital tract, and usually occurs just after the menstrual period. During menses, the cervical os is slightly open and the cervical mucous barrier is absent. Additionally, menstrual blood is an excellent *growth medium for* the pathologic organisms. The infection ascends from the vagina, through the cervical os to the uterus, Fallopian tubes, ovaries and occasionally the pelvic peritoneum. In most cases, the infection is polymicrobial: the tubal damage caused by *N. gonorrheae* or *C. trachomatis* renders the tubes more vulnerable to subsequent invasion and colonization by a variety of other organisms, including *Escherichia coli, Bacteroides* spp., *Ureaplasma* and *Mycoplasma*.

INCIDENCE AND RISK FACTORS

The Centers for Disease Control estimate that at least one million diagnosed cases of PID occur in the USA each year, in addition to the additional unrecognized infection of the tube[1]. It has been estimated that, in the USA, approximately 10–15% of women of reproductive age have had at least one episode of PID, and that about 30% of infertility and 50% of ectopic pregnancies are the direct sequelae of PID[2,3].

Risk factors for the development of salpingitis or PID include multiple sexual partners, age less than 25 years, history of previous salpingitis or PID, economic disadvantage, and intrauterine device use. Salpingitis may also occur after delivery, abortion or pelvic surgery.

CLINICAL FEATURES

Patients with PID present with a wide variation in clinical symptoms, including many women who will develop tubal damage without any symptoms of the disease. The Centers for Disease Control have recently suggested a new classification system for the disease, which includes: silent (asymptomatic) PID, atypical PID (minimal symptoms), acute PID (classic symptom complex) and PID residual syndrome (chronic). Generally, the affected patient presents with complaints of lower abdominal pain, fever, cervical discharge and occasionally menorrhagia. On physical examination, adnexal tenderness and tenderness with motion of the cervix and uterus are characteristic. High fever and peritonitis are more characteristic of gonococcal than non-gonococcal salpingitis, which is more likely to be clinically silent, therefore resulting in tubal damage secondary to delayed or inadequate diagnosis.

A minority of patients will have subacute salpingitis, complaining of vague lower abdominal pain only. On physical examination, there may be slight adnexal tenderness on cervical motion, but no presence of fever or rebound peritonitis.

DIAGNOSIS

Certainly history, physical examination and laboratory values are important in the diagnosis of PID; however, there is both a high false-positive rate and a high false-negative rate. Endocervical cultures positive for *N. gonorrheae* and *C. trachomatis* are definitive; culturing for other micro-organisms correlates poorly. The differential diagnosis includes lower genital tract infection, ovarian torsion or cyst rupture, appendicitis, ectopic pregnancy and endometriosis. Laparoscopy is the diagnostic procedure of choice, and is also extremely useful in the evaluation of the extent of tubal damage. Sonography has recently become an important diagnostic tool, as, unlike laparoscopy, it is non-invasive and well tolerated.

USE OF SONOGRAPHY IN THE DIAGNOSIS OF PID

Transabdominal sonography

Ultrasonography was identified early on as an important confirmatory tool in the diagnosis of tubo-ovarian abscess. Several retrospective studies[4-7] and one prospective study[8] have looked at the accuracy of transabdominal ultrasound in the diagnosis of pelvic abscesses secondary to pelvic inflammatory disease. Swayne and colleagues in 1984[9] first attempted to characterize the sonographic findings of PID using transabdominal probes. Patients with laparoscopically-confirmed PID underwent transabdominal sonography. Abnormal sonograms were classified into three groups: types I–III. Type I sonograms, the most uncommonly encountered group, contained cases where the sonographic abnormalities were related primarily to the uterus and sonographic signs of early endometritis, and no adnexal masses were present. Type II sonograms contained the presence of a focal extrauterine mass, usually in the adnexa, although these lesions were well defined. These masses were usually unilateral, ovoid, with variable internal architecture, and the average size was 5 cm. In 60%, the walls were sharp and smooth, the remainder having markedly irregular contours. Type III sonograms, the most frequently encountered group, represented a pelvic mass completely filled with a disorganized, heterogeneous echo pattern with solid and cystic areas, where the uterus could not be discretely identified in 36% of the cases. The sonographic–pathologic correlation was 70% for types II and III, and the group had one false-positive and ten false-negative diagnoses, usually when only early isolated tubal disease was present.

Transvaginal sonography

While transabdominal sonography was found to be reasonably useful as a confirmatory tool in the diagnosis of hydrosalpinx and tubo-ovarian abscess, the transabdominal appearance is often non-specific, and, in several studies, lacked consistent correlation to histopathological findings[7, 9]. Timor-Tritsch and Rottem first reported on the

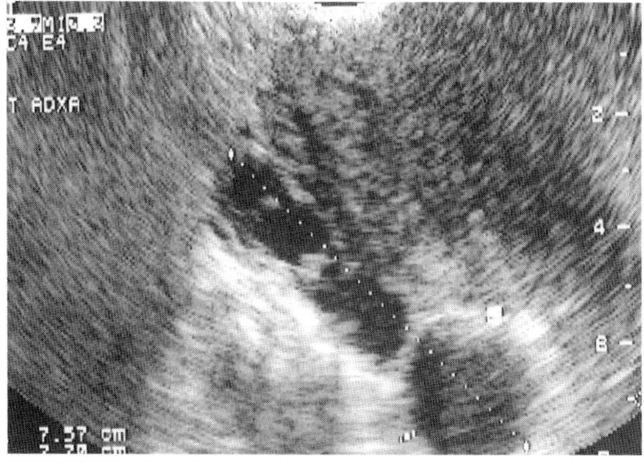
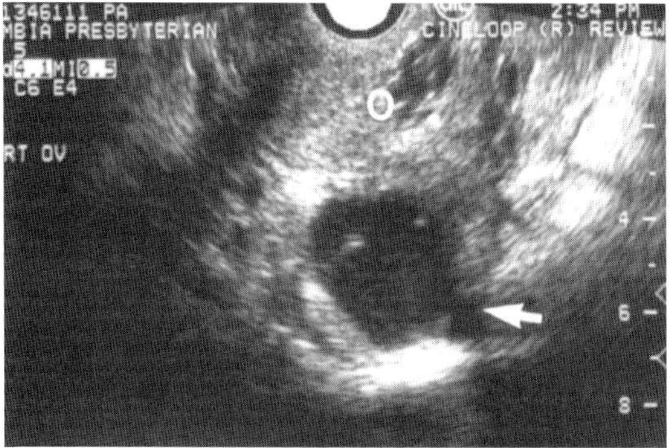

Figure 1 Acute hydrosalpinx: note the thick tubal walls. (Top panel) longitudinal section of the tortuous dilated Fallopian tube in the right adnexa; (bottom panel) cross-section of the tube, marked with the large arrow, above which the normal ovary (O) can be seen

use of transvaginal sonography in the study of the Fallopian tube in 1987[10]. The better resolution achieved with the higher frequency transvaginal probes revolutionized the study of the tube as a distinct entity. Although normal tubes are not often visualized, with the higher frequency probes, tubal walls, when filled with a contrasting fluid such as mucus or pus, are easily outlined. The diagnosis of a chronically damaged Fallopian tube can be made on serial scans in which the same sonographic picture is seen on subsequent examinations.

In a study by Bulas and colleagues published in 1992[11], transabdominal and transvaginal sonographic evaluations were compared in a population of adolescents with the clinical diagnosis of PID. The level of severity of PID, as determined at transabdominal sonography, was altered in 28 of 84 patients, with medical therapy changed in 23 of those cases because of additional transvaginal sonographic findings. Transvaginal sonography demonstrated superior anatomic detail over transabdominal sonography, and demonstrated abnormalities that were not seen at transabdominal sonography in 71% of patients.

SONOGRAPHIC SIGNS OF PELVIC INFLAMMATORY DISEASE

At the early stages of clinical PID there may be little or no sonographic changes seen within or adjacent to the Fallopian tubes, although occasionally a small amount of low-level echogenic fluid may be seen within the lumen or surrounding the fimbriated end. It is only in later stages of acute PID or chronic PID that a clearly delineated pelvic mass, known as tubo-ovarian complex or abscess, is seen.

Acute PID

As previously noted, early acute PID may have no detectable signs on transvaginal sonogram, except for a small fluid collection within the endometrial cavity or in the pelvis. In the Fallopian tubes an inflammatory response is initiated, resulting in edema, fluid accumulation, loss of normal tubal peristalsis and function, and the accumulation of purulent material. Pyosalpinges or hydrosalpinges are produced when an inflammatory process within the tube provokes a reaction causing adhesion formation, especially at the delicate fimbriated end. These adhesions then prevent normal circulation and removal of intraluminal secretions which, over time, distend the affected tube and create the fusiform shape typically characterized on sonography (Figure 1).

In the acute phase, the tubal wall is thick, and incomplete septae are seen (Figure 2). Low-level echogenic fluid, representing purulent exudate, may be seen within the thickened tube (Figures 3 and 4), and fluid levels are occasionally seen, corresponding to the dependent position. The typical sonographic picture of salpingitis, where there is evidence of tubal wall thickening and central hyperechoic mucosa with or without low-level echo-filled lumen, must not be confused with a sonographic picture of appendicitis. Terry and Forrest[12] describe a case of unilateral salpingitis confused with appendicitis; even once the specimens were removed, the size and appearance of

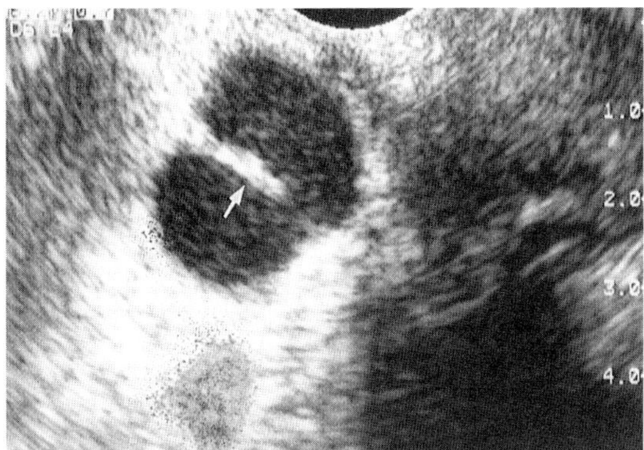

Figure 2 Cross-section of chronic hydrosalpinx with an incomplete septum (arrow). The incomplete septum is typical and instrumental to make this diagnosis. The low-level echogenic fluid filling the dilated tube is also evident

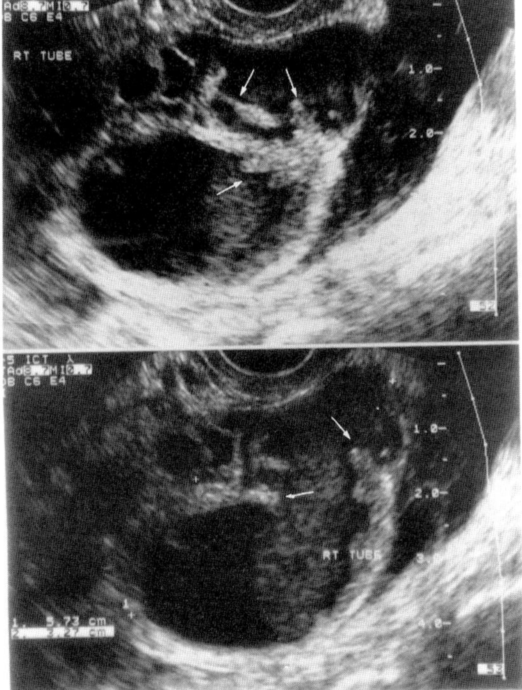

Figure 3 Acute salpingitis of the right tube. Note the distended fluid-filled and thick-walled right tube with the thickened salpingeal folds (arrows). The blocked tubes appear to be filled with material with low-level echogenicity, which may be consistent with pus. (Courtesy of Dr Z. Lebovitz, Bnai Zion Hospital, Haifa, Israel)

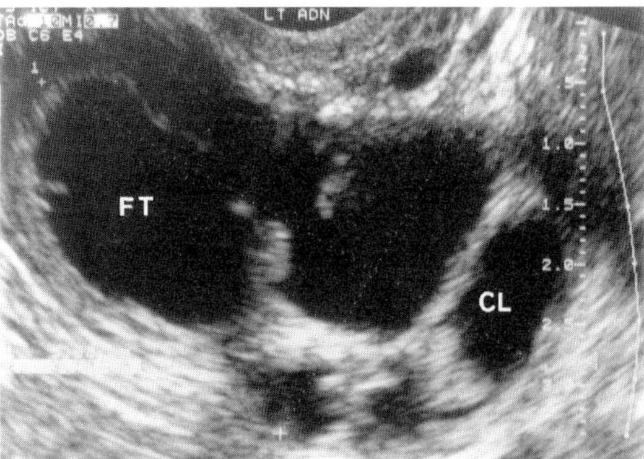

Figure 4 Acute pelvic inflammatory disease. The right adnexa is shown. At this stage of the acute process, it is still possible to discern the ovary with what appears to be the corpus luteum (CL) and the dilated thick-walled Fallopian tube (FT). (Courtesy of Dr Z. Lebovitz, Bnai Zion Hospital, Haifa, Israel)

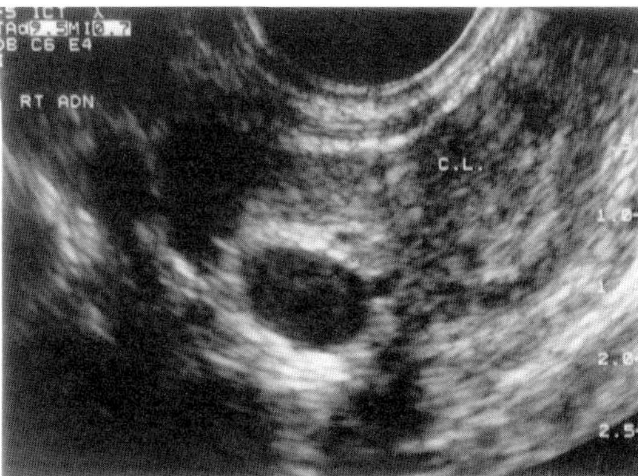

Figure 5 A differential diagnosis of adnexal findings. An increasing human β-chorionic gonadotropin level was seen in this patient who complained of right lower abdominal pain. A round lesion with hyperechoic walls and some low-level echogenic content of about 2×1.8 cm was seen in the right adnexa on the right side of the corpus luteum (CL). This lesion, marked by an arrow, was diagnosed as a non-live right ectopic pregnancy and treated with methotrexate. The differential diagnosis of this lesion is the cross-section of an acutely dilated right Fallopian tube

the inflamed salpinx were remarkably similar to the inflamed appendix on gross pathologic examination. Salpingitis must also be differentiated from ectopic pregnancy, as both disease processes share many etiologic and pathologic features (Figure 5).

A recent study by Patten and colleagues[13] prospectively analyzed preoperative transvaginal sonograms in women suspected of having acute PID and had a high degree of accuracy and sensitivity in predicting various findings. The sensitivity

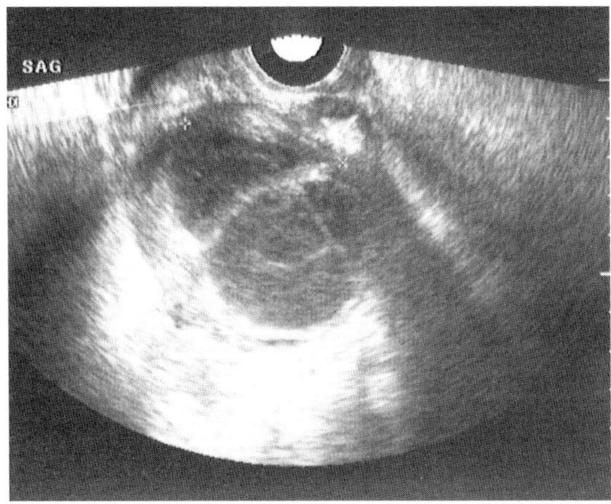

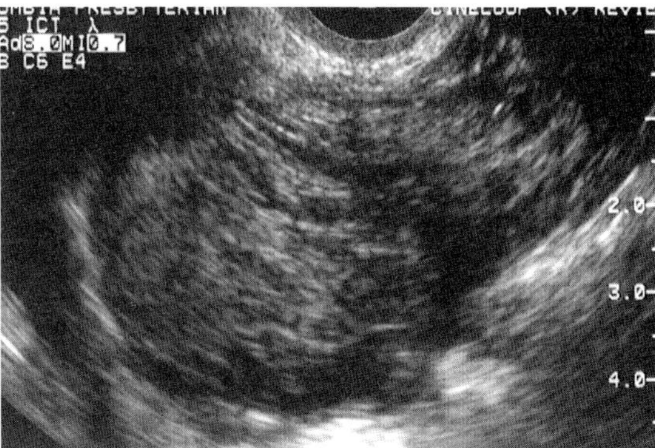

Figure 8 Tubo-ovarian abscess in the cul-de-sac. The independent structures can no longer be recognized: typical features of the tube or the ovaries cannot be found

Figure 6 An acute tubo-ovarian abscess on the right side involving the tube and ovary. Note that the normal anatomy of the ovary and/or the tube is no longer recognizable

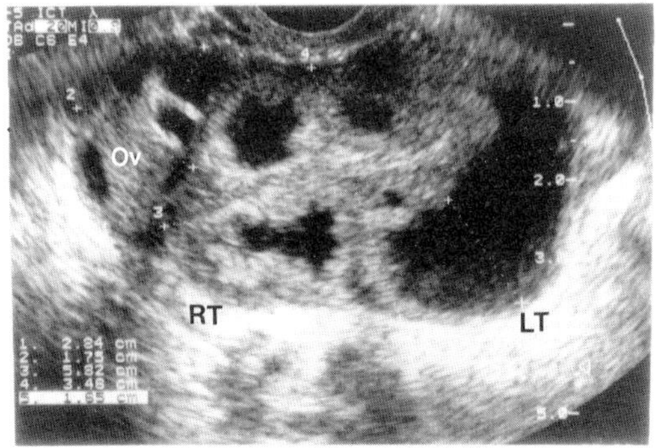

Figure 7 Acute pelvic inflammatory disease, bilateral tubal ovarian complex. Only the right ovary (Ov) is seen; however, three loops of the dilated right tube (RT) with the lumen appearing as the cog-wheel sign and the longitudinal section of the left tube (LT) are seen. In this stage of the disease, the different components of the lesions such as the ovaries and the tubes are still recognizable. (Courtesy of Dr A. Lebovitz, Bnai Zion Hospital, Haifa, Israel)

of transvaginal sonography for detecting tubal abnormalities was 93%, and ovarian/periovarian abnormalities was 90%. In contrast, transvaginal sonography was not a sensitive imaging technique in the detection of subtle uterine/periuterine abnormalities: only 25% of previously reported signs of endometritis, including indistinct endometrial stripe, ill-defined uterine contours and increased endometrial fluid, were identified. This group also found transvaginal sonography

insensitive for the detection of very small pelvic fluid collections, although quite sensitive once the pelvic fluid volume exceeded $20\,cm^3$.

Even in lower risk patients, that is, minimally symptomatic ambulatory patients with suspected PID, transvaginal sonography is accurate in the diagnosis of acute PID. A group from Finland concluded that a transvaginal sonogram suggestive of PID (a thickened fluid-filled tube with or without pelvic fluid) was found to have a sensitivity and a specificity of 85% and 100%, respectively[14]. These patients had a history of low abdominal pain, negative pregnancy test, and no gynecological procedures performed during the previous month, and endometrial biopsy revealing plasma cell endometritis was used as the criterion standard for acute PID. None of the patients with pelvic pain and normal sonograms had plasma cell endometritis. They conclude that transvaginal sonography performed well in the outpatient diagnosis of PID, and that, since a vast majority of patients with tubal infertility have no history of frank PID, use of this non-invasive modality is promising.

Tubo-ovarian abscesses or complexes represent a variety of findings and variable sonographic presentations, but the underlying common appearance includes a complex cystic and solid structure, which often does not allow for distinct identification of the tube or ovary (Figure 6). Tubo-ovarian abscesses or complexes may be seen in either the acute or chronic phase of PID, although they are considered to be the hallmark

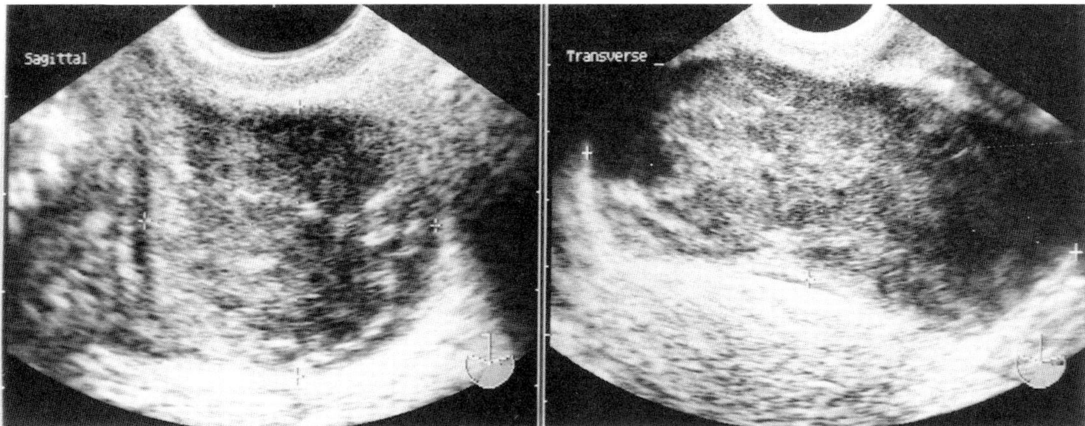

Figure 9 Hematoma formation in the cul-de-sac several days after transabdominal hysterectomy. At this stage, a $3 \times 5 \times 8$ cm mass of mixed echogenicity was found, which was tender at the touch of the transvaginal probe. Several days later this developed into an abscess. (Courtesy of Dr I. Schapiro, Bnai Zion Medical Center, Haifa, Israel)

of the severe acute PID episode. Although not found consistently, generally tubo-ovarian abscesses, more often than hydrosalpinges, have low-level internal echoes within the tube, representing pus, rather than simply endoluminal fluid, which is usually sonolucent. In severe and acute PID, large quantities of sonolucent or low-level echogenic pelvic fluid may be seen surrounding the complex mass, or in the cul-de-sac (Figures 7 and 8). Due to its non-invasive nature, transvaginal sonography is well suited to monitor clinical response to PID therapy via resolution of the sonographic findings over time. Pelvic abscesses may also develop postoperatively and appear sonographically as a typical tubo-ovarian abscess (Figure 9).

Timor-Tritsch and Rottem describe a typical appearance of the tubo-ovarian abscess using transvaginal sonography[10], which is similar to that described by Swayne's group transabdominally[9], although significantly more detailed structural analysis is obtained transvaginally. These authors prefer the term 'tubo-ovarian complex' to 'tubo-ovarian abscess' in describing the tortuous, dilated and fluid-filled Fallopian tube which 'embraces' the adjacent ovary. This ovary, therefore, cannot be well delineated although some ovarian follicles may still be present, enabling localization of the ovarian component of the mass (Figure 10).

The technique of vaginal color Doppler sonography has also recently been applied to the study of inflammatory tubal processes. Ten women with

tubo-ovarian infectious complexes caused by PID were investigated with vaginal Doppler sonography during the acute and healing phases of infection. Low-resistance blood flow was found at the margin of each infectious complex, the mean resistance index (RI) value was 0.5 and the mean pulsatility index (PI) value was 0.75. Once clinical resolution occurred, the corresponding RI and PI values were 0.63 and 1.17, respectively[15].

Chronic PID

The incidence of chronic PID has increased in proportion to the increasing rate of sexually transmitted diseases over the last 15 years. Recurrent PID is estimated to occur in up to 25% of patients, and the incidence of other sequelae, including risk of ectopic pregnancy, is even higher[16]. It is postulated that the microscopic tubal damage that occurs after one or more PID episodes retards tubal transport or entraps the fertilized embryo, resulting in tubal implantation.

The thin-walled hydrosalpinx is the sonographic hallmark of chronic PID (Figure 11). Obstruction of the fimbriated end of the tube results in a tubular structure with sonolucent fluid.

Hydrosalpinges produce the typical image of a homogeneous, elongated, fluid-filled mass, adjacent and usually medial to the ovary and often seen originating from the uterine cornu (Figure 12). The constant and non-peristaltic nature of the tube assists in differentiation of the diseased

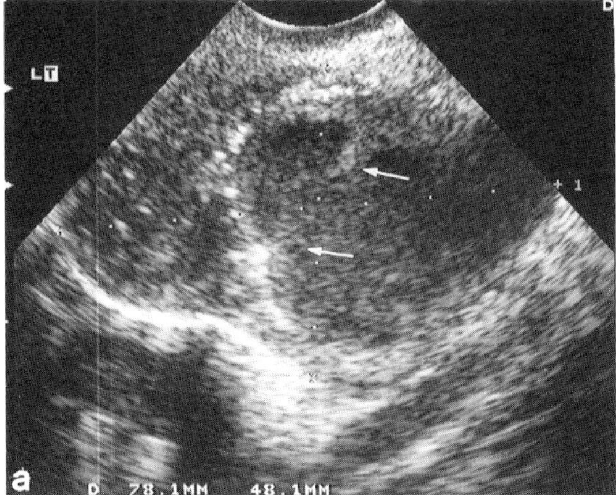

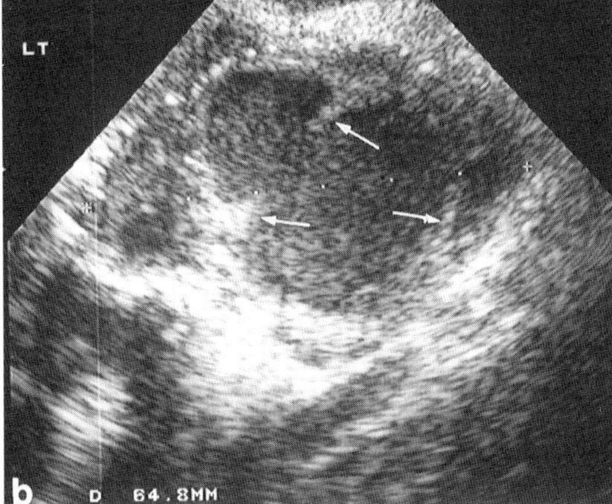

Figure 10 A 'full blown' inflammatory tubal ovarian complex, just before its transformation into tubal ovarian abscess. This is the acute stage of the disease. The size of this lesion is $7.8\times4.8\times6.4$ cm. (a), Longitudinal section; (b), transverse section of the lesion. Note that one could speculate that, on the left side of both pictures, the remnants of the ovaries are seen, while on the right side are the severely dilated tubes with incomplete septa (arrows). The remnants of endosalpingeal folds can be appreciated

tube from fluid-filled loops of small bowel. When the transducer probe is rotated 90° to scan the hydrosalpinx in the transverse plane, a specific sonographic pattern may be seen: 'cog-wheel'-like projections into the lumen of the fluid-filled tube, representing the endosalpingeal folds distorted by the luminal fluid (Figure 13). When the diseased tube is maximally distended by entrapped fluid, the endoluminal folds appear as small hypoechoic foci located on the luminal aspect of the tubal wall, described sonographically as 'beads on a

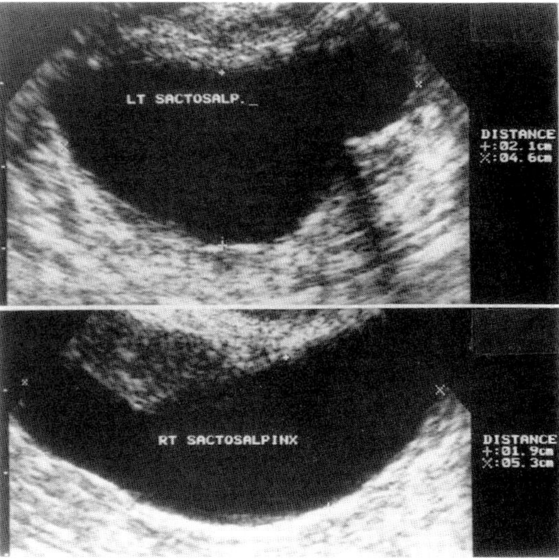

Figure 11 Two sections of chronic infection of the Fallopian tube. The top panel represents the left, the bottom panel, the right blocked fluid-filled hydrosalpinx. Note the thin walls and the almost total disappearance of the endosalpingeal folds. (Courtesy of Dr Z. Lebovitz, Bnai Zion Hospital, Haifa, Israel)

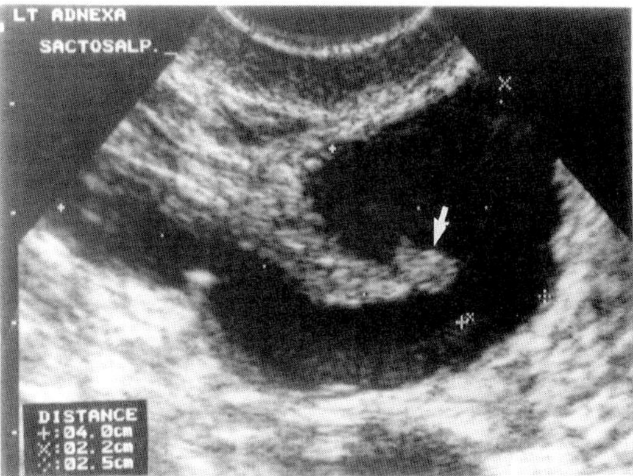

Figure 12 The typical appearance of sactosalpinx or blocked tube as a sequel of the chronic PID that the patient had several months prior. The typical incomplete septum (arrow) is pathognomonic and is the clue to the sonographic diagnosis of a chronically ill Fallopian tube. The walls are thin and, if the gain is increased, the tubal contents appear as of low-level echogenicity. (Courtesy of Dr Z. Lebovitz, Bnai Zion Hospital, Haifa, Israel)

string' (Figure 14). As in the more acute phase, incomplete tubal septae are seen, although the acute and chronic entities are easily distinguished by the thin, markedly distended tubal wall in chronic PID.

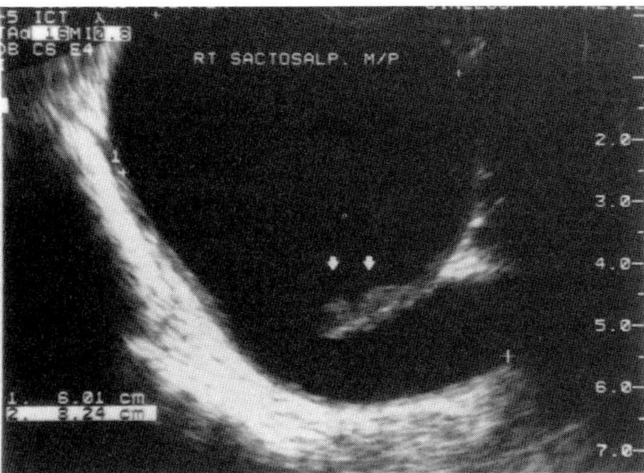

Figure 13 Chronic PID with a typical appearance of the retort-shaped, thin-walled right hydrosalpinx. The arrows point to the incomplete septa, which are the hallmark of this sonographic diagnosis. (Courtesy of Dr Z. Lebovitz, Bnai Zion Hospital, Haifa, Israel)

Other sequelae of chronic PID include pelvic adhesions and loculated fluid collections. These loculated collections are often incorrectly referred to as peritoneal inclusion cysts. Pelvic adhesions and pelvic inclusion cysts are thought to be responsible for many of the cases of chronic pelvic pain experienced by patients many years after their episode or episodes of PID. The sonographic loss of mobility of pelvic organs, most specifically the ovaries, suggests post-PID pelvic adhesions.

Timor-Tritsch and Rottem developed an important sonographic tool to identify pelvic adhesions, especially those secondary to infectious or inflammatory processes: the 'sliding organs sign'[10]. To elicit this sign, the transducer probe is pointed toward the pelvic organ or mass in question and a gentle push–pull movement, over several centimeters, is then begun. If no adhesions are present, the organ moves freely in the pelvis. If, for example, a tubo-ovarian mass is suspected, the relative positions of the tube, ovary and uterus are noted and do not change during the motion of the probe. This then presumes adherent association of the involved structures.

Pelvic inclusion cysts are not distinct cysts at all, but loculated pelvic fluid collections that are prohibited from normal unobstructed circulation patterns by pelvic adhesions, often resulting from chronic PID, and, less commonly, from previous pelvic surgery. They are easily confused with ovarian and paraovarian cysts, but may be differentiated sonographically by their constant appearance and persistence over time, and their irregular shapes which often conform to the contours of the abdomino-pelvic cavity (Figure 15).

TREATMENT OF PID

It is beyond the scope of this chapter to discuss treatment options in detail, but several aspects will be mentioned here. Certainly, intravenous antibiotics have been the mainstay of PID treatment

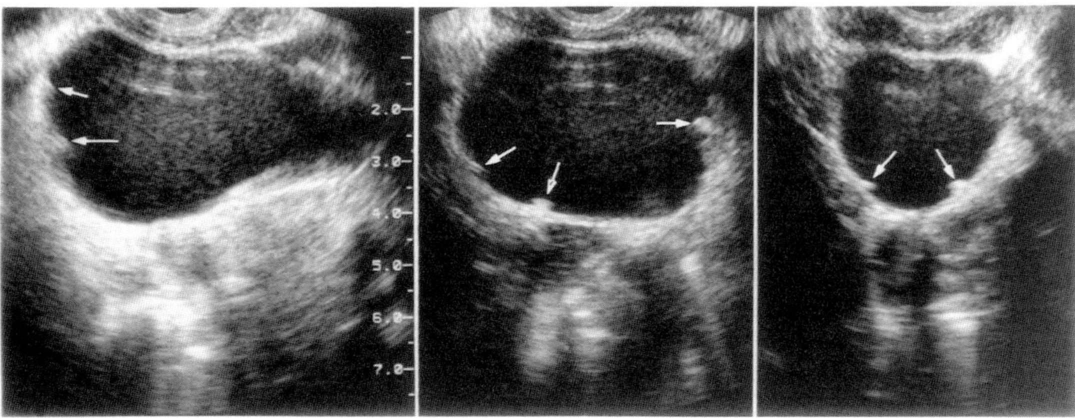

Figure 14 Chronic bilateral hydrosalpinx in a symptomless patient. Left panel, longitudinal section of the right tube; center panel, cross-section of the right tube; and right panel, cross-section of the left tube. Note that the fibrotic remnants of the endosalpingeal folds, resembling 'beads on a string', are marked by white arrows. (Courtesy of Dr Z. Lebovitz, Bnai Zion Hospital, Haifa, Israel)

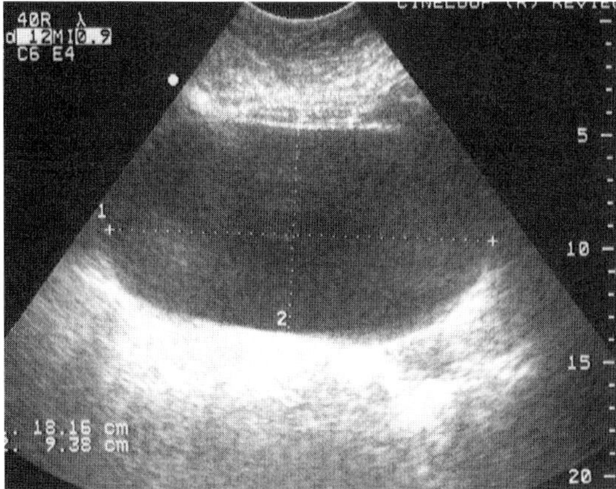

Figure 15 Peritoneal inclusion cyst. This transabdominal sonogram reveals a large unilocular peritoneal inclusion cyst. The anterior borders conform to the abdominal wall contour and there is no discernible cyst wall

in all patients, although, in a subset of patients, the presence of a pelvic abscess is so extensive that standard therapy fails. Laparotomy and laparoscopy are two modalities previously used for the treatment of pelvic abscesses and for lysis of adhesions. Although successful, these procedures are maximally invasive and pose anesthetic and surgical risks. Laparotomy for pelvic abscess is one of the most technically difficult surgical procedures that a gynecological surgeon performs[17]. There are several reports in the literature describing transabdominal[18] and transvaginal[19–21] sonographically directed percutaneous drainage of pelvic abscesses, and one study reporting success with computerized tomography-guided drainage in eight patients[22].

Because of the close proximity of the vaginal transducer probe to the pelvis and cul-de-sac, transvaginally guided puncture of pelvic abscesses is ideally suited. A needle can be directed alongside the shaft of the vaginal transducer and inserted into pelvic collections under direct sonographic observation (Figure 16). Under continuous observation, the fluid may be safely aspirated, and the needle can then be subsequently aimed and replaced into the various loculations sequentially. At the end of the procedure, the needle may simply be removed, or a plastic catheter may be placed to be left to drain continuously for several days. The two-step pelvic fluid drainage and catheter placement technique is especially suited to pelvic abscesses refractory to traditional antibiotic therapy. First, the abscess is drained using a 14-gauge needle, then a flexible guide wire is introduced through the needle. The needle is extracted, leaving the wire in place, and a plastic catheter with multiple perforations is slid over the guide wire. The guide wire is then pulled and the indwelling pelvic catheter is fixed to the patient's thigh, where it remains in place for approximately 2–4 days, or until there is no further drainage of fluid. The patient is rescanned prior to catheter removal and subsequently as clinically necessary. The procedure is technically easy, has little morbidity, and high patient tolerance.

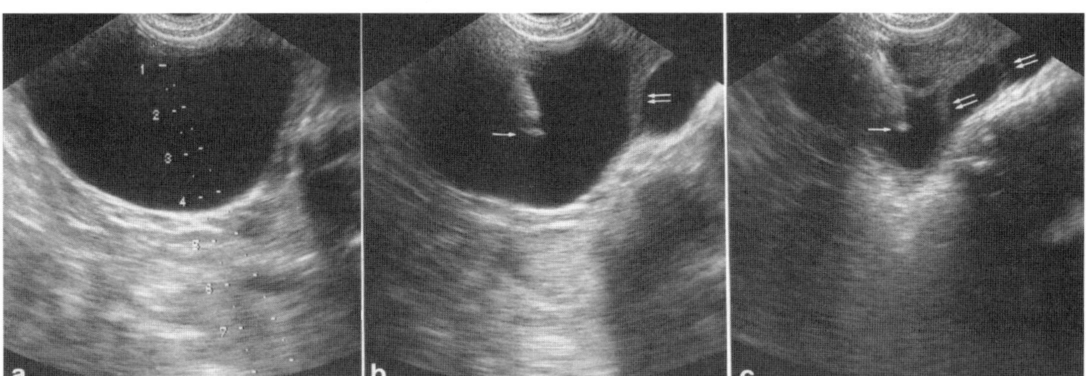

Figure 16 Transvaginally-guided drainage of a peritoneal inclusion cyst. (a) Peritoneal inclusion cyst with a needle guide superimposed on the sonographic image; (b) the tip of the inserted needle is marked with a single arrow. The typically appearing pelvic adhesions are marked with double arrows, separating the loculated fluid compartments; and (c) withdrawal of pelvic fluid continues under direct sonographic visualization. The needle tip is again marked by a single arrow, pelvic adhesions by double arrows

SUMMARY

Salpingitis secondary to PID is one of the two most commonly encountered tubal disorders, the other being ectopic pregnancy. With the increasing incidence of sexually transmitted diseases, tubal damage secondary to delayed diagnosis or incomplete treatment is a serious concern. Transvaginal sonography is both sensitive and accurate in diagnosing inflammatory and infectious changes in the Fallopian tube, including hydrosalpinx and tubo-ovarian complexes. The better resolution obtained with the higher frequency transvaginal probes allows for identification of distinct tubal architecture and subtle abnormalities not appreciated with the transabdominal approach. Transvaginal sonography can easily be performed in the setting of acute PID as a diagnostic adjunct to laparoscopy, and also used to monitor clinical resolution of more extensive disease once therapy has been instituted. Transvaginal sonography also has a role in the work-up of a patient with unexplained infertility, where sonographic evidence of a hydrosalpinx or pelvic adhesions and loculated fluid imply previously unknown PID. Transvaginal sonography is well suited to the evaluation of inflammatory processes of the Fallopian tube since the consistent presence of fluid in these disease entities permits superior tubal visualization.

References

1. Centers for Disease Control (1985). *C. trachomatis* infections: policy guidelines for prevention and control. *Morbidity and Mortality Weekly Report*, **34** (3, suppl.), 53s–74s
2. Gales, W. and Wasserheit, J.N. (1991). Genital chlamydial infections: epidemiology and reproductive sequelae. *Am. J. Obstet. Gynecol.*, **164**, 1771–81
3. Expert committee on pelvic inflammatory disease (1991). Research directions for the 1990s. *Sex. Trans. Dis.*, 1846–64
4. Filly, R.A. (1979). Detection of abdominal abscesses: a combined approach employing ultrasonography, computed tomography, and gallium-67 scanning. *J. Assoc. Can. Radiol.*, **30**, 202
5. Taylor, K.J.W. De Graaft, M.C.I., Wasson, J.F., Rosenfield, A.T. and Audriole, V.T. (1978). Accuracy of grey scale ultrasound diagnosis of abdominal and pelvic abscesses in 220 patients. *Lancet*, **1**, 83
6. Uhrich, P.C. and Sanders, R.C. (1976). Ultrasonic characteristics of pelvic inflammatory masses. *J. Clin. Ultrasound*, **4**, 199
7. Spirtos, N.J., Bernstine, R.L., Crawford, W.L. and Fayle, J. (1982). Sonography in acute pelvic inflammatory disease. *J. Reprod. Med.*, **27**, 312–20
8. Golden, N., Cohen, H., Gennari, G. and Neuhoff, S. (1987). The use of pelvic ultrasonography in the evaluation of adolescents with pelvic inflammatory disease. *Am. J. Dis. Child.*, **141**, 1235–8
9. Swayne, L.C., Love, M.B. and Karasick, S.R. (1984). Pelvic inflammatory disease: sonographic-pathologic correlation. *Radiology*, **151**, 751–6
10. Timor-Tritsch, I.E. and Rottem, S. (1987). Transvaginal ultrasonographic study of the fallopian tube. *Obstet. Gynecol.*, **70**, 424–8
11. Bulas, D.I., Ahlstrom, P.A., Sivit, C.J., Blask, A.R.N. and O'Donnell, R.M. (1992). Pelvic inflammatory disease in the adolescent: comparison of transabdominal and transvaginal sonographic evaluation. *Radiology*, **183**, 435–9
12. Terry, J. and Forrest, T. (1989). Sonographic demonstration of salpingitis: potential confusion with appendicitis. *J. Ultrasound Med.*, **8**, 39–41
13. Patten, R. M., Vincent, L.M., Wolner-Hanssen, P. and Thorpe, E. Jr. (1990). Pelvic inflammatory disease: endovaginal sonography with laparoscopic correlation. *J. Ultrasound Med.*, **9**, 681–9
14. Cacciatore, B., Leminen, A., Ingman-Friberg, S., Ylostalo, P. and Paavonen, J. (1992). Transvaginal sonographic findings in ambulatory patients with suspected pelvic inflammatory disease. *Obstet. Gynecol.*, **80**, 912–16
15. Tinkanen, H. and Kujansuu, E. (1993). Doppler ultrasound findings in tubo-ovarian infectious complex. *J. Clin. Ultrasound*, **21**, 175–8
16. Droegemueller, W. (1987). Upper genital tract infections. In Droegemueller, W., Herbst, A.L., Mishell, D.R. Jr., and Stenchever, M.A. (eds.) *Comprehensive Gynecology*, pp. 614–42. (St. Louis: C.V. Mosby Company)
17. Weisenfeld, H.C. and Sweet, K.L. (1993). Progress in the management of tuboovarian abscesses. *Clin. Obstet. Gynecol.*, **36**, 433–44
18. Worthen, N.J. and Gunning, J.E. (1986). Percutaneous drainage of pelvic abscesses: management of tuboovarian abscesses. *J. Ultrasound Med.*, **5**, 551–6
19. Nelson, A.L., Sinow, R.M., Renslo, R., Renslo, M.J. and Atamede, F. (1995). Endovaginal ultrasonographically guided transvaginal drainage for treatment of pelvic abscesses. *Am. J. Obstet. Gynecol.*, **172**, 1926–35

20. van Sonnenberg, E., D'Agostino, H.B., Casola, G., Goodacre, B.W., Sanchez, R.B. and Taylor, B. (1991). Ultrasound-guided transvaginal drainage of pelvic abscesses and fluid collections. *Radiology*, **181**, 53–6

21. van der Kolk, H.L. (1991). Small deep pelvic abscesses: definition and drainage guided with an endovaginal probe. *Radiology*, **181**, 283–4

22. Tyrrel, R.T., Murphy, F.B. and Bernardino, M.E. (1990). Tubo-ovarian abscesses: CT-guided percutaneous drainage. *Radiology*, **175**, 87–9

Doppler studies of the vascularity of the Fallopian tube

F. A. Aleem

INTRODUCTION

The Fallopian tubes are paired muscular organs which extend from the uterus to the ovaries. They serve as a path for the ova into the uterine cavity and for fertilization following ovulation. Both Fallopian tubes are covered with peritoneum, except in the infundibular region where there is communication between the tube and the abdominal cavity. The oviducts are prone to bacterial infection, and consequences are acute and chronic salpingitis, hydrosalpinx, abundant adhesions around the tubes, ectopic pregnancy and infertility. Until the introduction of transvaginal high-frequency probes for the assessment of the female pelvic anatomy, sonographic reports rarely, if ever, referred to the Fallopian tube, and Fallopian tube pathology was generally related to ectopic pregnancy. However, it is now obvious that a significant part of adnexal pathology, described ultrasonically as multilocular or cystic-solid masses, is caused by chronic tubal inflammatory disease. The ultrasonic appearance of the pathologically changed tubes as multilocular structures with irregular walls and septa, suspicious papillary projections and clear to dense content may lead to the false-positive detection of malignant or benign ovarian lesions. Therefore, it is important to establish and categorize tubal ultrasonic anatomy, pathology and vascularity. Distinguishing accurately tubal from ovarian vascularity might help to discriminate and detect neovascular signals in cases of ovarian malignancy.

FALLOPIAN TUBE ANATOMY

The human oviduct is a tubular, seromuscular organ attached distally to the ovary and proximally to the lateral aspect of the uterine fundus, and is supported lengthwise by the mesosalpinx. The oviduct's length is 7–12 cm and may vary individually. Based on morphologic and anatomic differences, the oviduct is divided into four segments: the infundibulum, whose fimbriated end surrounds the tube's distal ostium; the ampullary region; the isthmic portion; and the intramural or interstitial portion, which is contained within the wall of the uterus[1].

FALLOPIAN TUBE VASCULARITY

The oviduct's arterial blood supply is derived from two main sources: the uterine and ovarian arteries (Figure 1). The uterine artery near the cornu sends a branch to supply the interstitial portion of the tube and the cornu. It then splits into two trunks (about 2 cm below the tubal origin)[2], one of which supplies the medial portion of the tube and anastomoses with the tubal branches from the ovarian artery, while the other branch anastomoses with the ovarian artery branches which supply the ovary. The anastomosis in the broad ligament can be extensive[1,2]. However, three types of the oviduct vascularization (Figure 2) can be distinguished[3]: Type I (60%), observed most frequently, where tubal branches of the uterine artery and the ovarian artery are of similar size, and therefore, the organ vascularization originates in an equal degree from both arteries; Type II (35%), where the tubal branch of the uterine artery is the main vessel of the Fallopian tube, its external diameter being at least twice as large as the tubal branch arising from the ovarian artery; and Type III, which occurs most rarely (5%); in this variation the ovarian artery is the main supplying artery not only for the ovary and the Fallopian tube, but for the fundus and the uterine body.

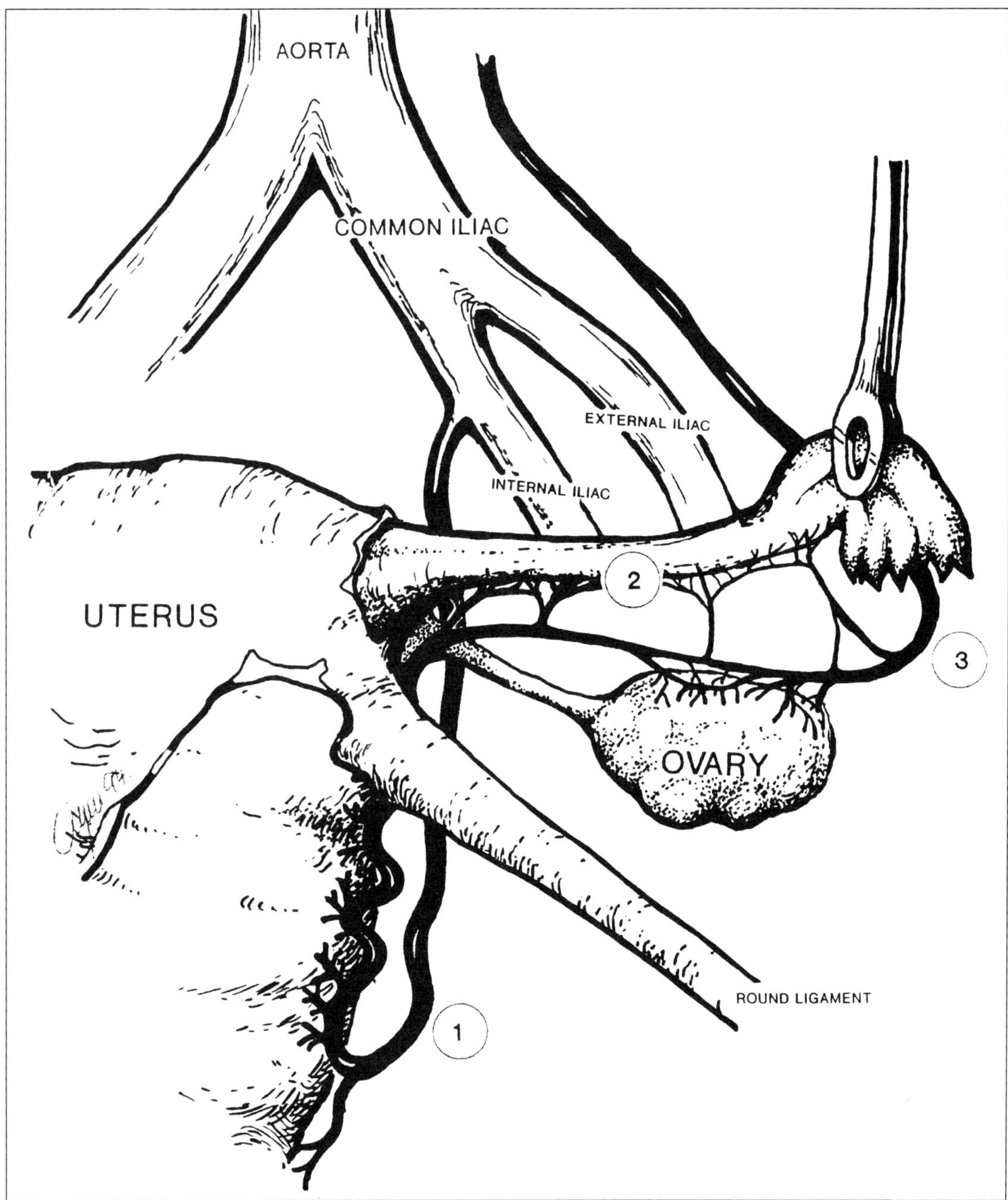

Figure 1 Schematic presentation of pelvic arteries: uterine artery (1); tubal arteries (2); main ovarian artery in the infudibulopelvic ligament (3)

The diameter of the tubal arteries has been measured, following injection of the tubes with epoxy resins, by sectioning blocks from tubal tissue with a diamond saw[4]. The mean diameter of the main uterine artery, before its branching on the ascending and descending branches, is 2.4 mm

(Figure 3). The diameter of the ascending branch gradually decreases towards its end and anastomoses with the main ovarian artery. The mean diameter of the main ovarian artery is 1.6 mm. These two arteries give tubal branches whose diameters vary from 0.3 mm at the isthmic end to

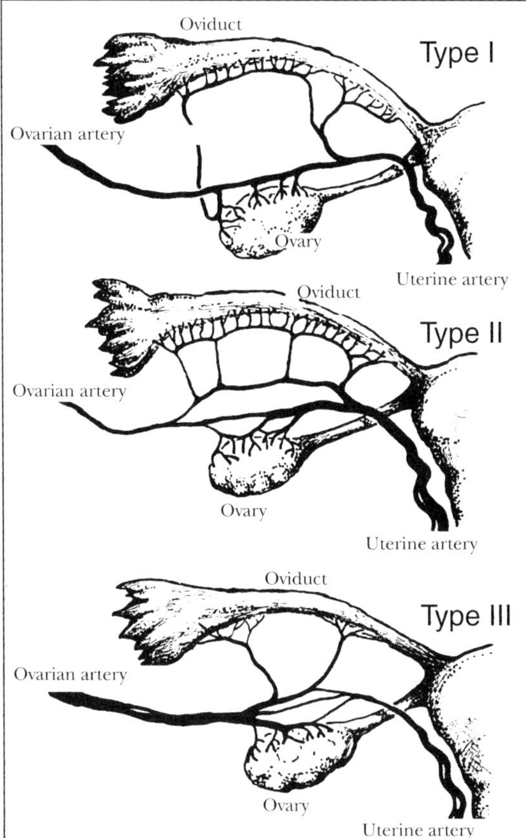

Figure 2 Schematic presentation of the different origins of the tubal artery. Type I, tubal branches of the uterine and the ovarian artery are of similar size; Type II, tubal branch of the uterine artery is the main vessel of the Fallopian tube; Type III, the ovarian artery is the main tubal artery supplying both the ovary and the Fallopian tube

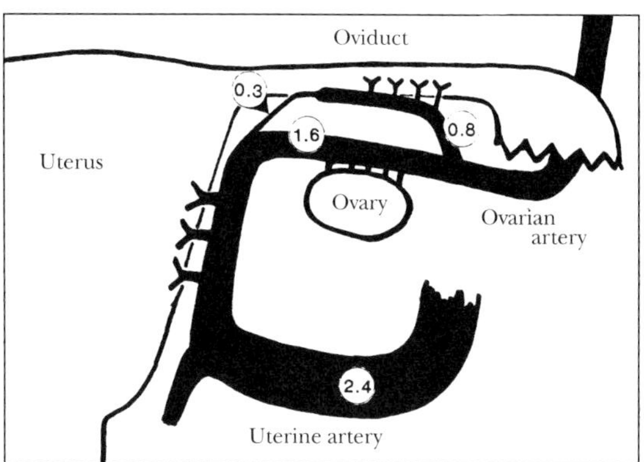

Figure 3 Schematic presentation of the pelvic vessel mean diameters in mm

0.8 mm at the ampullar part of the tube. There is a significant difference in the diameter of the main uterine and ovarian arteries between pre-menopausal and postmenopausal women. The mean diameter of these arteries in postmenopausal women is smaller by almost 1 mm in comparison with the diameter of the same arteries in the premenopausal woman. However, such a large difference in vessel diameter has not been noted in the case of tubal arteries, which vary only by 0.2–0.3 mm. Fallopian tubes of women in the reproductive phase of life receive their blood supply mainly from the ovarian artery, while Fallopian tubes of postmenopausal women predominantly receive their blood supply from the uterine artery[4].

According to histological investigations of the Fallopian tube vascular bed during various phases of the menstrual cycle and during early intra-uterine pregnancy, isolated mechanisms of blood shunting in cyclic changes of the Fallopian tube's functional activity have been noted[5]. The blood shunting is formed by the occlusive arterioles and arterio-venular semi-shunts situated, mainly, in the tubular isthmus[5]. Intimal cushions, muscular-elastic constrictors, valves and other regulating mechanisms of the bloodstream are contained in the mucosal layer[6]. The mucosal tunic is only one part of the microcirculatory bed of the uterine tube, which is presented by serous, subserous, muscular and mucosal plexuses. The main pathways for the transportation and distribution of blood to the corresponding parts of the tube are sector arteries, which are situated in the subserous tela along the anterior and posterior semicircles of the organ, and originate from the uterine and ovarian arteries' tubal branches[6].

ULTRASONOGRAPHIC APPEARANCE OF THE FALLOPIAN TUBE

Until the introduction of vaginal probes, the Fallopian tube was considered to be practically undetectable by ultrasonography. The *normal* tiny Fallopian tube, lying between the uterus, bowels and ovary or hidden in the cul-de-sac, also could be missed with high-frequency probes. The normal-sized Fallopian tube is not seen by trans-vaginal sonography, unless surrounded by fluid.

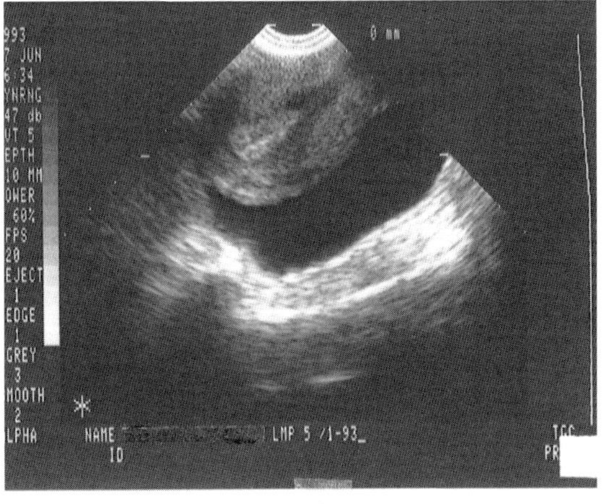

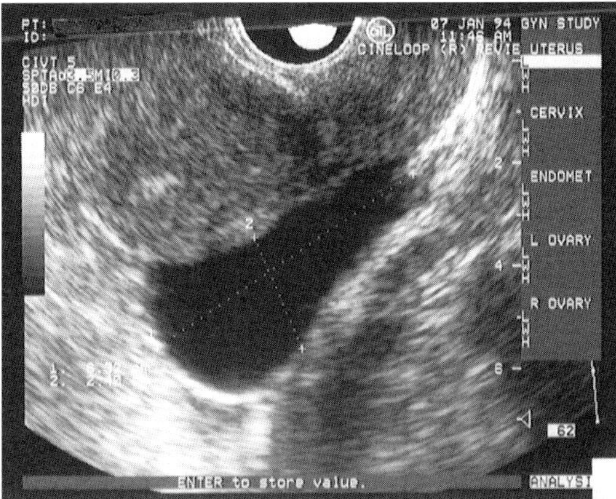

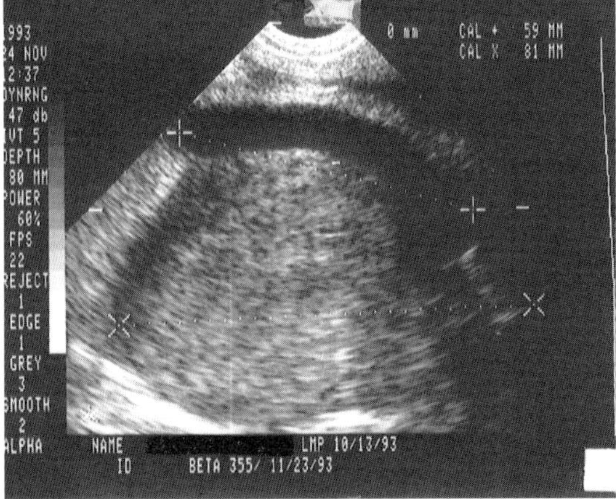

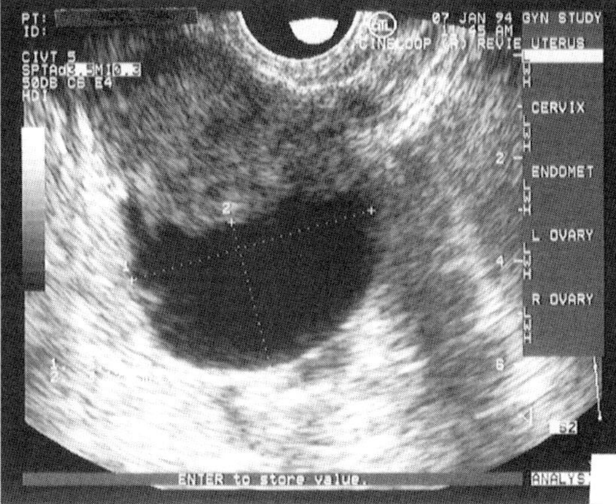

Figure 4 Transvaginal image of hydrosalpinx. Top panel, unilocular cyst with irregular walls located behind and adherent to the uterus; bottom panel, tubular cystic structure surrounding uterine fundus

Figure 5 Other examples of unilocular cystic structures with irregular walls and no intracystic echoes. Hydrosalpinx was confirmed at the laparoscopy

This contrasting fluid may be serous fluid present in the pelvis of healthy patients, follicular fluid present during or after ovulation, blood, ascitic fluid, or products of an exudative or infectious process[7]. If outlined by fluid, the normal Fallopian tube presents as a tortuous, 1-cm wide echogenic structure. The tube's lumen cannot be detected unless it is filled with fluid. Therefore, the pathologic tube is more easily recognizable, even without contrasting pelvic fluid. The Fallopian tube wall may appear thin and over-stretched when a contrasting fluid fills the lumen, as in the case of a sactosalpinx, hydrosalpinx or tubo-ovarian abscess, or when thickened in several inflammatory processes or tubal malignancy. *Hydrosalpinx* produces the image of a dilated tube that contains a homogeneous sonolucent fluid (Figures 4 and 5). The fluid that is secreted distends the tube, resulting in a fusiform anechoic adnexal mass. The tapered fusiform shape and lack of peristalsis of a hydrosalpinx usually allows its differentiation from fluid-filled small bowel loops. Sometimes, a dilated tube will have fluid content with the appearance of two distinct fluid levels: one sonolucent and the other, a weakly echoic material, representing the pus[8]. In the case of hydrosalpinx, the pathologic tube will often reveal the sonographic image of a simple or multi-locular ovarian or paraovarian cyst (Figure 6). However, when hydrosalpinx is presented as a complex mass with thick walls, septae, suspicious papillary projections and/or mixed echogenic structure, incorrect conclusions could be drawn (Figure 7).

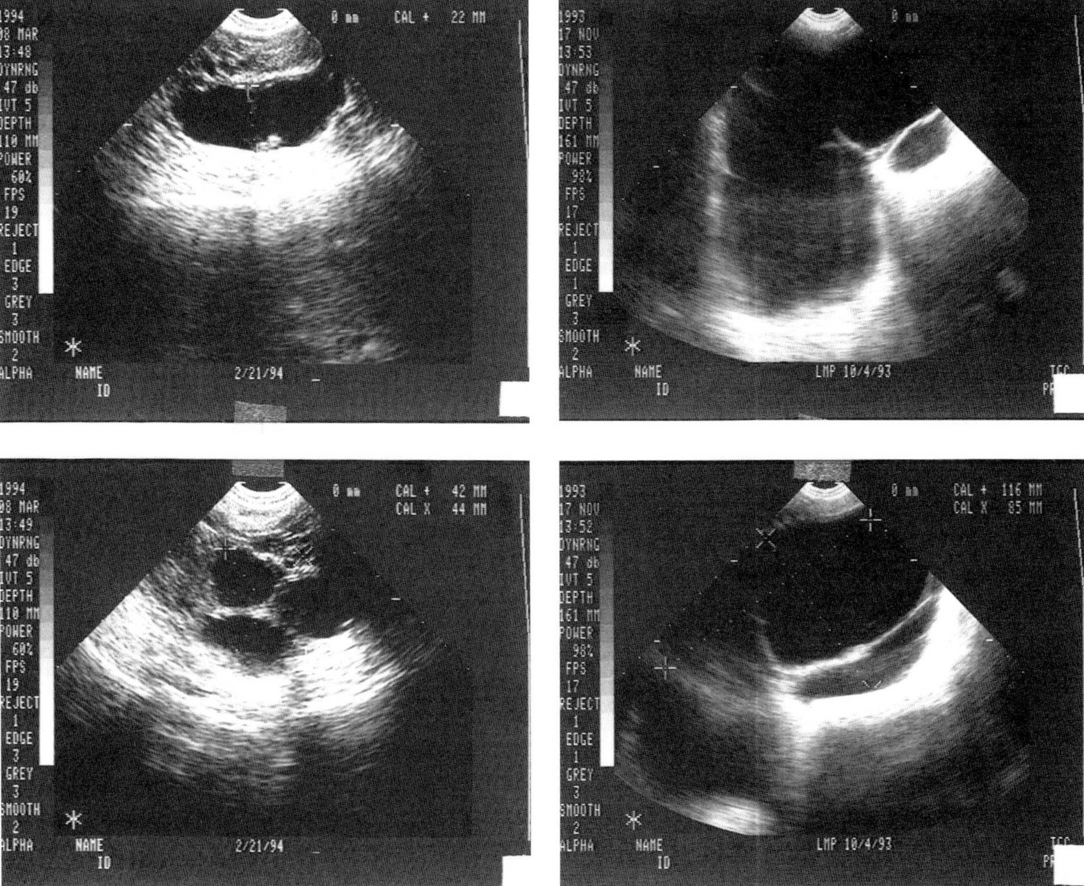

Figure 6 Hydrosalpinx. Top panel, bilocular cystic structure with thin septa, located adherent to the uterus; bottom panel, trilocular cystic structure with thin septa and no intracystic echoes

Figure 7 Multilocular appearance of the huge hydrosalpinx. Longitudinal (top panel) and transverse (bottom panel) scans of the cystic structure reveal thin septa and no intracystic echoes

Tubo-ovarian abscess appears as tortuous, irregular structures that appear to be adherent to the ovary. It is sometimes difficult to differentiate, on the basis of ultrasonography, a simple hydrosalpinx, which does not involve the ovary, from a tubo-ovarian abscess. The presence of follicles within the ovary may help the recognition and identification of an ovarian component of the tubo-ovarian abscess.

Table 1 Blood flow characteristics of pathologic Fallopian tube in terms of color and pulsed Doppler

	Fallopian tube pathology		Index	
Reference	Malignant	Benign	RI	PI
Shalan *et al.* [31]	1	—	0.34	—
Tekay and Jouppila [26]	—	3 TOA	0.60	0.90
Kurjak *et al.* [20]	—	3 TOA	0.62	—
Timor-Tritsch *et al.* [25]	—	3 HYS	0.68	1.30
	—	2 TOA	0.70	1.50
Schneider *et al.* [28]	—	2 HYS	1.0	—
Carter *et al.* [29]	1	—	NDA	NDA

RI, resistance index; PI, pulsatility index; TOA, tubo-ovarian abscess: HYS, hydrosalpinx: NDA, no data available

Tubal pregnancy can be diagnosed with high accuracy based on the presence of an intact tubal gestational sac, and/or associated fluid or blood clots in the pouch of Douglas, decidual reaction and history of amenorrhea followed by uterine bleeding. However, the morphological description and vascular characteristics of the ectopic pregnancy are described in other chapters.

In the case of tumors of the Fallopian tube, primary *malignant tumors* comprise fewer than 1% of all malignancies of the female genital tract[9], while secondary tumors are more common. Carcinoma of the Fallopian tube is the most common form of primary tubal malignancy, and ultrasonically is presented as a solid adnexal mass or as a complex solid-cystic mass[10,11]. It is obvious that tubal pathology is very difficult to differentiate from ovarian pathology when complex masses are found. Sassone and colleagues[12] in a comprehensive study of the sonographic appearance of ovarian masses prospectively identified only three of the 23 tubal pathologies. Lerner and associates[13] published sonographic data about eight cases of hydrosalpinges and five tubo-ovarian masses. The authors used a morphological score with a cut-off value of 3. The mean score was 1.3 for hydrosalpinges and 4 for the tubo-ovarian masses. Most of the tubo-ovarian masses found were assessed as malignant lesions. These data reveal the difficulty in obtaining accurate morphological assessment of the tubal pathology, because of mistakes frequently made in establishing tubal pathology as ovarian, and because of the bizarre morphology – these tubal conditions are erroneously recognized as malignant adnexal lesions. However, a simple procedure may be applied in these instances to distinguish the Fallopian tube from an adnexal mass. The transcervical injection of sterile saline or ultrasound contrast agent may be used to outline oviducts, which will only float in the free fluid[14–16] if the oviducts are patent. The same procedure may also be used for the assessment of patency of the oviducts.

PULSED AND COLOR DOPPLER SONOGRAPHY OF THE FALLOPIAN TUBE

The introduction of color Doppler and its promising results in discriminating between benign and malignant adnexal lesions[17–19] has helped significantly in improving sonographic specificity. It has become possible to visualize and characterize different tissue vascularities and to assess accurately blood flow profiles.

It is well known that malignant tumors are rich in neovascularization[17–19]. These new vessels are often bizarre in architecture, rich in arteriovenous anastomoses with a diminished resistance to blood flow. Doppler assessment of resistance to blood flow is aided by the addition of color flow imaging, which allows rapid guidance of the pulsed Doppler spectral analysis of the studied vessels. Some investigators, by using pulsed color Doppler, have presented promising results in the differentiation between benign and malignant pelvic masses with high sensitivity and specificity[20–25], while others have found significant overlapping in the values of resistance index (RI) or pulsatility index (PI) between benign and malignant adnexal lesions[26–30]. There is the possibility that the divergent data and disagreements over color and pulsed Doppler sonography values may be due to a lack of equipment standardization. Also, the transvaginal color Doppler technique depends on the ultrasonographer's skills and knowledge. In order to reduce the ultrasonographer's subjectivity during the color Doppler imaging, it is necessary to standardize the following parameters: color pulse repetition frequency (PRF), PRF range, output power, the lowest velocities used and specific characteristics of the different pelvic vessels. These are a few of the technical and protocol requirements which should be standardized.

Generally, benign tubal lesions are poorly vascularized with high to moderate impedance to blood flow (Color plates 8–13). From previously mentioned publications[20, 25, 26, 28, 29, 31], the blood flow characteristics of benign tubal lesions are presented in Table 1. Mean PI and RI values calculated from Table 1 are 1.23 and 0.74, respectively. In this study, only one case of tubal adenocarcinoma was published with color and pulsed Doppler characteristics[31]. It was presented as a complex adnexal mass, richly vascularized with low impedance to blood flow, with RI of 0.34. Currently, there is no overlap of RI or PI results between this malignant case and the aforementioned reported benign tubal lesions. However,

Table 2 Continuous Doppler flow indices of the tubal and ovarian arteries (reproduced from Aleem *et al.*[32], with kind permission)

Type of vessel	n	RI			PI		
		Mean	SE	Range	Mean	SE	Range
Tubal artery	34	0.59	0.02	0.28–0.95	1.11	0.09	0.45–2.57
Ovarian artery (IPL)	35	0.73	0.02	0.28–0.91	1.53	0.10	0.37–2.79
Ovarian artery (hilum)	12	0.58	0.03	0.37–0.78	1.03	0.11	0.51–1.83

RI, resistance index; PI, pulsatility index; IPL, infundibulopelvic ligament

difficulty exists in recognizing and discriminating tubal benign masses from ovarian lesions, such as those described by Sassone and colleagues[12] and Lerner and associates[13]. Therefore, the possibility of increased overlapping in blood flow data in adnexal masses could be caused by either unrecognized or missed tubal pathology or even tubes with a normal vascular network. If a normal or pathologic tube is fused with an ovary, then the tubal vessel may be mistaken for the ovarian vessel. This hypothesis requires proof that normal tubal vascularity may mimic a neovascular blood flow signal during transvaginal Doppler examinations. The solution to this problem can be found in a continuous Doppler study, where the probe would be placed directly over the tubal and/or other adnexal vessels intraoperatively and the Doppler signals recorded.

CONTINUOUS DOPPLER OF FALLOPIAN TUBE VESSELS

Recently, our group presented a study[32] to characterize the Doppler flow signals from the ovarian artery in the infundibulo-pelvic ligament (IPL), the ovarian branch in the hilum and the tubal artery. This goal was achieved by using a continuous wave Doppler intraoperatively (Multigon Industries, Inc, Mt. Vernon, USA). A total of 24 patients undergoing laparotomy for benign gynecological disorders (18 patients with uterine myomas; one case of cervical pathology; three patients with pelvic adhesions and two patients with mild endometriosis without adnexal masses) were included in the study. Twenty-one (87.5%) of our patients were premenopausal and three (12.5%) were postmenopausal.

In a total of 24 patients, 34 recordings of tubal arteries (Figure 8), 12 ovarian hilum arteries and 35 ovarian arteries (IPL) were demonstrated and recorded (Table 2). Arteries from each adnexa were considered as a single group during analysis of the data. No significant difference was found when flow indices of the right and left side vessels (tubal, IPL and hilar arteries) were compared in the same patient. The mean RIs for the tubal and ovarian IPL artery were 0.59 ± 0.02 and 0.73 ± 0.02, respectively. The mean PIs for the tubal and ovarian artery (IPL) were 1.11 ± 0.09 and 1.53 ± 0.1, respectively. The tubal artery showed significantly lower RI and PI when compared to the ipsilateral ovarian artery at the infundibulopelvic ligament ($p < 0.001$ and $p = 0.002$, respectively) and its hilar branches ($p = 0.03$ for RI and $p = 0.03$ for PI).

It was concluded that tubal artery flow signals, which have been measured directly for the first time in this study, are characteristic and are distinct from the ovarian artery signals. The tubal artery is in close proximity to the ovary and it is difficult to identify the normal Fallopian tube by transvaginal sonography. This makes misinterpretation of signals from the tubal vessels during transvaginal color Doppler sonography as signals from the ovarian vessels a possibility to consider. Mixing between signals during transvaginal color Doppler sonography might be a source of confusion, especially during screening of normal adnexa. Some of the low-resistance signals detected in the adnexal region during transvaginal scanning of the ovaries might be picked up from surrounding vessels (tubal arteries) and may not necessarily mean a neovascularization. Also, sampling ovarian vessels at different levels

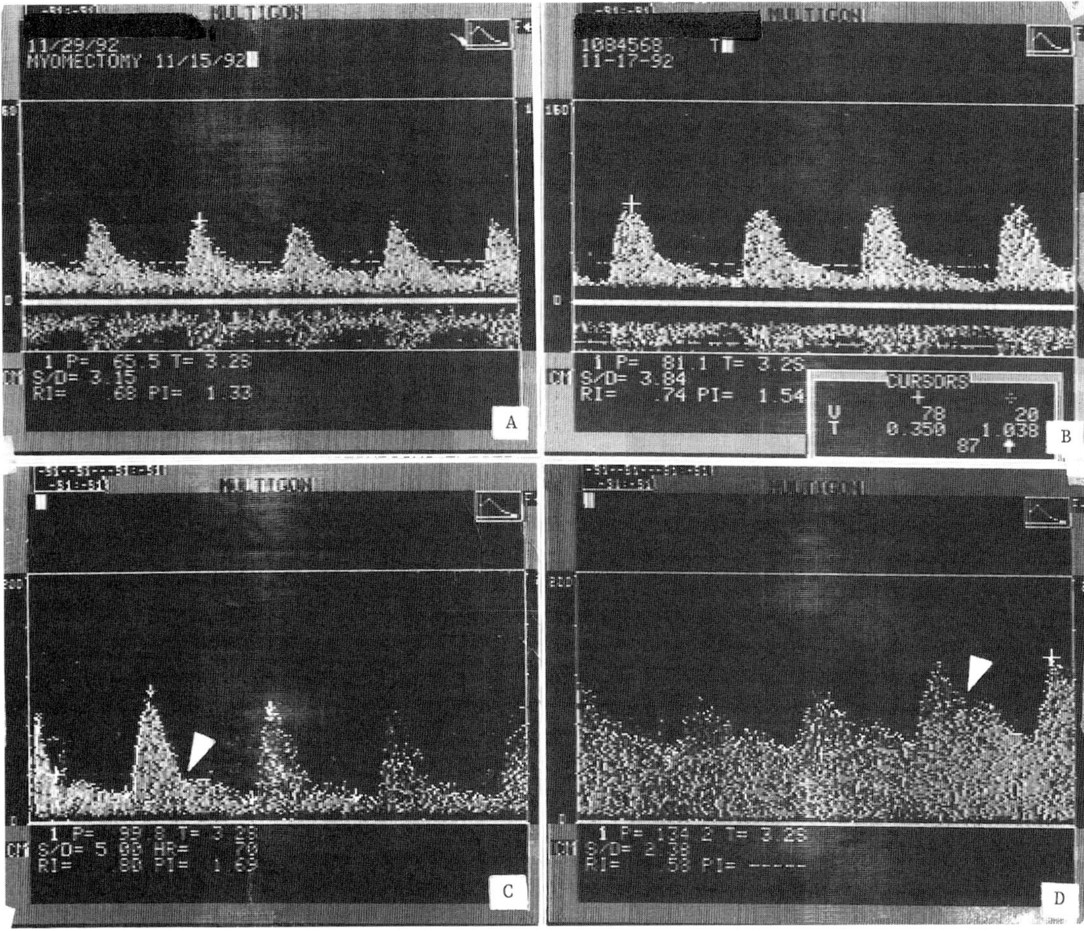

Figure 8 Continuous Doppler flow signals obtained from the tubal artery. Top panels, left and right, Doppler sonograms show moderate to high vascular impedance to blood flow; bottom panels, left and right, show increased vascular impedance to blood flow; an early diastolic notch (arrow) can be seen. Note that end-diastolic flow is increased on the bottom right-hand sonogram

(IPL or hilar regions) might significantly affect the obtained RI and PI, and might explain some of the discrepancies in the reported data from different institutions. Recognition of the flow signal from the tubal artery may help to differentiate ovarian and tubal vessels detected during color Doppler sonography.

SUMMARY

To date, vascularization of the Fallopian tube has been described only for tubal microsurgery purposes, but that knowledge was neglected in the assessment of the adnexal vascularity in terms of transvaginal color and pulsed Doppler examination. Tubal arteries have cyclic menstrual changes in their vascular impedance to blood flow, probably due to blood shunting performed by the occlusive arterioles and arterio-venular semi-shunts situated, mainly, in the Fallopian tube isthmus. As a consequence, an abnormal blood flow pattern with low vascular impedance can be detected with transvaginal color Doppler. If abnormal morphology of the adnexa is involved, tubal arteries may be mistaken for peripheral ovarian arteries and recognized as a neovascular 'malignant' signal. It seems that tubal vascularity may influence our beliefs about adnexal vascularity as well as our understanding of blood flow hemodynamic changes in normal and abnormal adnexal conditions.

References

1. Eddy, C.A. and Pauerstein, C.J. (1980). Anatomy and physiology of the Fallopian tube. *Clin. Obstet. Gynecol.*, **23**, 1177–93

2. Kjer, J.J. and Mogensen, A.M. (1989). The arterial supply of the parametrium. *Eur. J. Obstet. Gynecol. Reprod. Biol.*, **30**, 275–8

3. Wydrzynski, M. and Sikorski, A. (1989). Anatomical examinations of the tubal arteries for the needs of gynecological microsurgery. *Folia Morphol. (Warsz.)*, **48**, 219–29

4. Brokelmann, J. (1989). Funktionelle Morphologie des Eileiters. *Arch. Gynecol. Obstet.*, **245**, 391–5

5. Glukhovets, B.I., Lebedev, S.S. and Ukhov, Y.I. (1982). Peculiarities of the Fallopian tube vascular bed in women. *Arkhiv Anatomii, Gistologii i Embrilogii*, **82**, 51–5

6. Vakalyuk L.M., Zelyak, V.L. and Melman, E.P. (1988). The blood bed of the human uterine tube. *Arkhiv Anatomii, Gistologii i Embriologii*, **94**, 86–93

7. Timor–Tritsch, I.E. and Rottem, S. (1987). Transvaginal ultrasonographic study of the Fallopian tube. *Obstet. Gynecol.*, **70**, 424–8

8. Fleischer, A.C. and Entman, S.S. (1992). Differential diagnosis of pelvic masses. In Chervenak, F.A., Issacson, G.C. and Campbell, S. (eds.) *Ultrasound in Obstetrics and Gynecology*, Vol. II, pp. 1643–53. (Boston: Little, Brown)

9. Morley, P. and Hollman, A.S. (1992). Gynecologic malignancy. In Chervenak, F.A. Isaacson, G.C. and Campbell, S. (eds.) *Ultrasound in Obstetrics and Gynecology*. Vol. II, pp. 1739–76. (Boston: Little, Brown)

10. Subramanyam, B.R., Raghavendra, B.N., Whalen, C.A. and Yee, J. (1984). Ultrasonic features of Fallopian tube carcinoma. *J. Ultrasound Med.*, **3**, 391–3

11. Zarbo, G., Giardinella, S. and Nardo, F. (1986). Primary adenocarcinoma of the Fallopian tube. *Eur. J. Gynecol. Oncol.*, **7**, 217–20

12. Sassone, A.M., Timor-Tritsch, I.E., Artner, A., Westhoff, C. and Warren, W.B. (1991). Transvaginal sonography characterization of ovarian disease: evaluation of a new scoring system to predict ovarian malignancy. *Obstet. Gynecol.*, **78**, 70–6

13. Lerner, J.P., Timor-Tritsch, I.E., Federman, A. and Abramovich, G. (1994). Transvaginal ultrasonographic characterization of ovarian masses with an improved, weighted scoring system. *Am. J. Obstet. Gynecol.*, **170**, 81–5

14. Stern, J., Peters, A. and Coulam, C.B. (1992). Color Doppler ultrasonography assessment of tubal patency: a comparison study with traditional techniques. *Fertil. Steril.*, **58**, 897–900

15. Allahbadia, G.N. (1992). Fallopian tubes and ultrasonography: the Sion experience. *Fertil. Steril.*, **58**, 901–7

16. Deichert, U., Schlief, R., van de Sandt, M. and Daume, E. (1992). Transvaginal hysterosalpingo-contrast sonography for the assessment of tubal patency with gray scale imaging and additional use of pulsed wave Doppler. *Fertil. Steril.*, **57**, 62–7

17. Kurjak, A., Zalud, I., Jurkovic, D., Alfirevic, Z. and Miljan, M. (1989). Transvaginal color Doppler for the assessment of pelvic circulation. *Acta Obstet. Gynecol. Scand.*, **68**, 131–4

18. Bourne, T.H., Campbell, S., Steer C., Whitehead, M.I. and Collins, W.P. (1989). Transvaginal color flow imaging: a possible new screening technique for ovarian cancer. *Br. Med. J.*, **299**, 1367–70

19. Fleischer, A.C., Rodgers, W.H., Rao, B.K., Keppler, D.M., Worrel, J.A., Williams, L. and Howard, W.J. (1991). Assessment of ovarian tumor vascularity with transvaginal color Doppler sonography. *J. Ultrasound Med.*, **10**, 563–8

20. Kurjak, A., Schulman, H., Sosic, A., Zalud, I. and Shalan, H. (1992). Transvaginal ultrasound, color flow and Doppler waveforms of the post-menopausal adnexal mass. *Obstet. Gynecol.*, **80**, 917–21

21. Bourne, T.H., Campbell, S., Reynolds, K.M., Whitehead, M.I., Hampson, J., Royston, P., Crayford, T.J.B. and Collins, W.P. (1989). Screening for early familial ovarian cancer with transvaginal ultrasonography and colour blood flow imaging. *Br. Med. J.*, **306**, 1025–9

22. Fleischer, A.C., Rodgers, W.H., Kepple, D.M., Williams, L.L. and Jones, III H.W. (1993). Color Doppler sonography of ovarian masses: a multi-parameter analysis. *J. Ultrasound Med.*, **12**, 41–8

23. Kawai, M., Kano, T., Kikkawa, F., Maeda, O., Ogichi, H. and Tomoda, Y. (1992). Transvaginal Doppler ultrasound with color flow imaging in the diagnosis of ovarian cancer. *Obstet. Gynecol.*, **79**, 163–7

24. Weiner, Z., Thaler, I., Beck, D., Rottem, S., Deutsch, M. and Brandes, J.M. (1992). Differentiating malignant from benign ovarian tumors with transvaginal color flow imaging. *Obstet. Gynecol.*, **79**, 159–62

25. Timor-Tritsch, I.E., Lerner, J.P., Monteagudo, A. and Santos, R. (1993). Transvaginal ultrasonographic characterization of ovarian masses by means of color flow-directed Doppler measurements and a morphologic scoring system. *Am. J. Obstet. Gynecol.*, **168**, 909–13

26. Tekay, A. and Jouppila, P. (1992). Validity of pulsatility and resistance indices in classification of adnexal tumors with transvaginal color Doppler ultrasound. *Ultrasound Obstet. Gynecol.*, **2**, 338–44

27. Hata, K., Hata, T., Manabe, A., Sugimura, K. and Kitao, M. (1992). A critical evaluation of transvaginal Doppler studies, transvaginal sonography,

magnetic resonance imaging, and CA125 in detecting ovarian cancer. *Obstet. Gynecol.*, **80**, 922–6

28. Schneider, V., Schneider, A., Reed, K.L. and Hatch, K.D. (1993). Comparison of Doppler with two-dimensional sonography and CA125 for prediction of malignancy of pelvic masses. *Obstet. Gynecol.*, **81**, 983–8

29. Carter J., Saltzman, A., Hartenbach, E., Fowler, J., Carson, L. and Twiggs, L.B. (1994). Flow characteristics in benign and malignant gynecologic tumors using transvaginal color flow Doppler. *Obstet. Gynecol.*, **83**, 125–30

30. Valentin, L. and Sladkevicius, P. (1993). Limited contribution of Doppler velocimetry to the differential diagnosis of extrauterine pelvic tumors. *Ultrasound Obstet. Gynecol.*, **3** (Suppl. 1), 21

31. Shalan, H., Sosic, A. and Kurjak, A. (1992). Fallopian tube carcinoma: recent diagnostic approach by color Doppler imaging. *Ultrasound Obstet. Gynecol.*, **2**, 297–9

32. Aleem, F., Zeitoun, K., Calame, R., Trinca, D., Zalud, I. and Schulman, H. (1995). The characterization of flow signals from tubal and ovarian arteries using intraoperative continuous wave Doppler. *Ultrasound Obstet. Gynecol.*, **4**, 304–9

The diagnosis of benign and malignant tumors of the Fallopian tube 8

A. Kurjak, F. Bonilla-Musoles and S. Kupešić

INTRODUCTION

The preoperative ultrasonic diagnosis of benign or malignant tumors of the Fallopian tubes presents one of the greatest challenges for the sonographer. This is particularly so in the reliable diagnosis of primary tubal carcinoma, a tumor which is one of the rarest malignancies of the female genital tract. Fewer than 1% of primary gynecological cancers are tubal in origin and, in a review of nine population-based cancer registries in the United States between 1973 and 1984, the average annual incidence was 3.6/1000000 women. It is therefore not surprising that the diagnosis is only infrequently made preoperatively. Early diagnosis is made by chance and usually in patients who were undergoing tubal sterilization. The disease occurs more often in women of low parity with an average age of 52 years. The triad of pain, vaginal bleeding and leukorrhea is considered pathognomonic of tubal carcinoma. Some authors report primary infertility in more than 50% of investigated patients. Postmenopausal vaginal bleeding is the most common symptom and therefore one must seriously consider the diagnosis of Fallopian tube carcinoma when the dilatation and curettage (D&C) is negative for carcinoma of the endometrium and the symptoms persist.

BENIGN TUMORS OF THE FALLOPIAN TUBE

Although the muscles of the Fallopian tube and the uterus are of the same embryologic origin (Müllerian ducts), leiomyomas of the Fallopian tube are as exceptional (fewer than 100 cases have been reported) as those of the uterus (the most common tumor found in woman) are usual. Leiomyomas of the Fallopian tube are commonly incidental findings, as they are asymptomatic and small. However, there are reported cases of large tubal myomas associated with acute abdomen consequent to its torsion[1].

Tubal pregnancy associated with tubal leiomyomas, in which the tubal myoma was the obstructing factor, have also been reported[1–3].

None of these few cases of tubal leiomyomas described in the literature were diagnosed preoperatively. In our case, transvaginal color flow Doppler was an aid to establish the diagnosis of a primary benign tumor of the Fallopian tube. To the best of the authors' knowledge, this is the first report of a leiomyoma of the Fallopian tube diagnosed preoperatively. We will therefore describe our case in detail.

Case history

A 38-year-old woman, gravida 2, para 1, with an unremarkable past history was referred to the gynecological department in Valencia due to right lower quadrant tenderness for the past 6 months. Pelvic examination was unspecific.

Transvaginal color Doppler sonography was carried out (Aloka color Doppler SSD-680 EX scanner with a 5-MHz transvaginal probe). Sonographic examination revealed a solid right adnexal mass 20×18 mm. The adnexal mass was separated from the uterus as well as the ovary on the same side, and seemed to be an integral part of the right Fallopian tube (Color plate 14). Color flow velocity waveform studies revealed a high-resistance flow with resistance index (RI) 0.72 and a pulsatility index (PI) 1.81 (Color plate 15). A primary benign tumor of the Fallopian tube was suspected. On explorative laparotomy, a solid nodule was found in the isthmus of the right

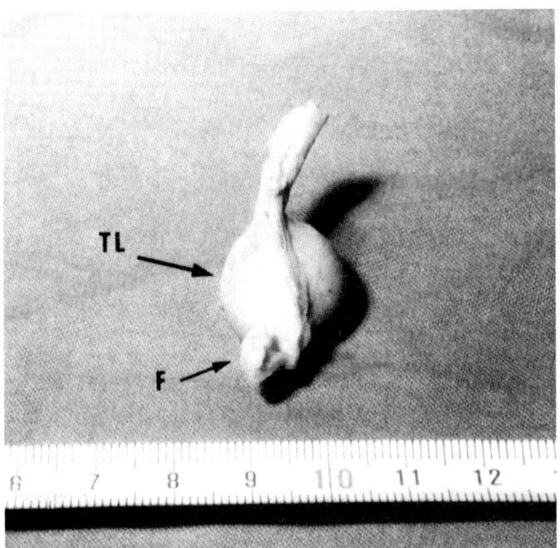

Figure 1 Pathological specimen showing a Fallopian tube leiomyoma (TL) located at the isthmus of the tube (F)

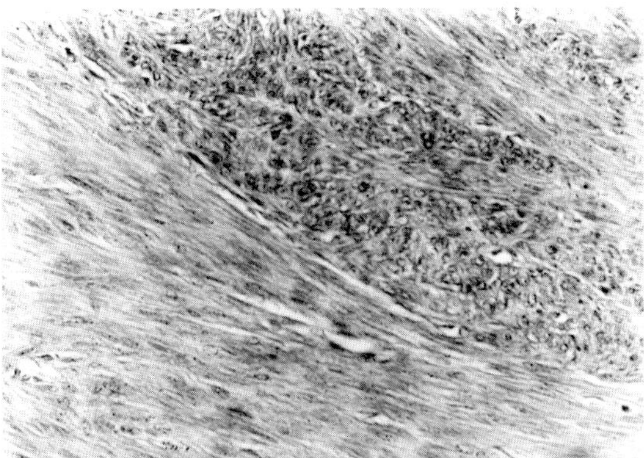

Figure 2 Microscopic examination shows bundles of smooth muscle cells with spindle nuclei without degeneration

Fallopian tube (Figure 1). A right salpingectomy was performed. The pathological examination revealed the presence of a $16 \times 14 \times 14$ mm subserous tubal leiomyoma (Figure 2).

MALIGNANT MASSES

Until recently, preoperative diagnosis for malignant masses of Fallopian tubes did not exist; it was rather a matter of chance than the triumph of any scientific diagnostic method. In a remarkable review of 376 cases of tubal carcinoma, McGoldrick and colleagues[4] found only one diagnosed correctly preoperatively. More recently, Eddy and colleagues[5] analyzed the data of 74 patients regarding tubal malignancies and only two cases of tubal carcinoma were diagnosed correctly before surgery. Podratz and his group[6] in 1986 detected only three cases of tubal cancer out of 47 patients studied.

Ayhan and colleagues[7] reported a study of eight cases of primary Fallopian tube carcinoma. These patients constituted 0.3% of all gynecological malignancies encountered during the study period. The most common symptom was abnormal vaginal bleeding (four patients). All patients but one had extra-tubal disease at the time of surgery. No patient was operated with a preoperative diagnosis of tubal cancer.

Dava and colleagues[8] described six *adenocarcinomas* of the Fallopian tube that resembled the female adnexal tumor of probable Wolffian origin. The tumor, which occurred in patients from 38 to 66 years of age (average 55 years), typically formed intraluminal masses. One was an incidental finding on the microscopic examination. Microscopically, the tumors were characterized by a predominant pattern of small, closely packed cells punctured by numerous glandular spaces, which were typically small but occasionally were cystically dilated. Many of the glands contained a dense colloid-like secretion that was positive when treated with the periodic acid-Schiff stain. Small amounts of intracellular mucin were present in all cases. In the solid areas of three cases, spindle cells, that focally formed concentric whorls, were present. In all cases small numbers of tubular glands, typical of endometrioid adenocarcinoma, were identified. The cytologic atypia and mitotic activity of the tumors were variable, but they exceeded what is usually seen in Wolffian duct tumors. The authors stressed the need to differentiate this unusual form of endometrioid adenocarcinoma from a tumor of Wolffian duct origin.

Soundara and associates[9] published a review of Fallopian tube carcinoma over 20 years. Nine cases of tubal carcinoma were found among approximately 9000 gynecological malignancies. Most patients were diagnosed as having malignant ovarian tumor, but two cases presented unusually, one as Meig's syndrome and another as acute hemoperitoneum. The often-stressed symptom of discharge of *hydrops tubae profluens* could not be elicited in any patient. All patients underwent surgical treatment and radiotherapy or chemotherapy.

Malignant mixed Müllerian tumor of the Fallopian tube has also been described. Chiou and colleagues[10] wrote that only 37 cases of this extremely rare neoplasm with a poor prognosis have been reported up to date. A case is reported of malignant mixed Müllerian tumor of the Fallopian tube occurring in a 63-year-old woman who presented with postmenopausal vaginal spotting for 7 months. In another paper, Chang and colleagues[11] found a similar incidence of the malignant mixed Müllerian tumor of the Fallopian tube. They reviewed the case of a 66-year-old female who had complained of profuse watery vaginal discharge for 1 month. Vaginal cytology in that patient was positive for malignancy while the endometrial curettage and cervical biopsies were both negative. Gynecological sonography revealed a left adnexal mass 6 cm in diameter. She underwent exploratory laparotomy after complete oncologic work-up. The main tumor was confined to one tube but the cytology of the peritoneal washing was positive for cells typical of adenocarcinoma. Carcinomatosis peritonei occurred 12 months after the primary surgery and she died 1 month later.

The similarities of Fallopian tube carcinoma and ovarian carcinoma have been described by Tokunaga and co-workers[12] in 1991. Tubal carcinoma and serous adenocarcinoma of the ovary were found to be remarkably similar in their biological characteristics and tumor markers, which suggests that the basis for the management of tubal carcinoma and that of ovarian carcinoma could be similar.

The cases with rare histologic features, including endometrioid carcinoma, mixed Müllerian tumor, and malignant fibrous histiocytoma have been reported.

Rosen and colleagues[13] studied the incidence and prognostic factors of primary carcinoma of the Fallopian tube in a retrospective multicenter study of 115 cases during the period 1980–1990. Stages were classified according to the modified FIGO system for ovarian cancer; grading followed the criteria of Hu and colleagues[14]. The mean age of the patients was 62.5 years. Forty-seven (40.9%)

tumors were found to be in stage I, 20 (17.4%) in stage II, 34 (29.6%) in stage III and 14 (12.1%) in stage IV. In 82 patients, the tumor could be completely removed. The surgical method applied in 95 patients was a removal of the uterus, the adnexa, and/or omentum, or the lymph nodes. Postoperatively, patients underwent adjuvant therapy which was either irradiation or chemotherapy. The 5-year survival rate for all stages was 36.5%. In stages I and II, the 5-year survival rate was 50.8% compared to 13.6% in stages III and IV. FIGO stages I and II and a residual tumor less than 2 cm in advanced disease had a prognostically favorable impact, which was proven in univariate as well as multivariate analysis.

Unfortunately, there is no high index of suspicion for tubal malignancy, although more than 80% of patients have pelvic mass detected before surgery. In a certain number of cases, cervical cytology, X-ray films of the pelvis, computed tomography or hysterosalpingography are usually no more specific than the pelvic examination. Roberts and Lifshitz[15] in 1982 analyzed 102 cases and pointed out that carcinoma of the tube was seen often in early, and more curable stages. More than 50% of the patients with Fallopian tube malignancy reported recently were diagnosed during stage I or II, which compares much more favorably to those patients with ovarian cancer in which 70–80% had stage III or IV disease when the diagnosis was established.

Nearly all malignacies of the tube are adenocarcinomas and bilaterality has been noted in 10–25% of the patients. Tumors are usually large and therefore detectable by pelvic examination, although the smallest reported adenocarcinoma measured 2.3 mm. It seems impossible to detect such a small lesion by bimanual pelvic palpatation.

Sedlis[16] in 1978 found that the 5-year survival rate for all cases of tubal carcinoma was 38% regardless of stage. Other authors have noted 5-year survival rates as high as 88% in stage I Fallopian tube carcinoma. In fact, prognosis mimics ovarian carcinoma when stage is used as a discriminating factor.

Fallopian tube sarcoma is extremely rare – only 30 such cases have been reported. One patient with stage Ia survived longer than 5 years[17]. Most patients are in their sixth decade of life and of low parity.

Undoubtedly, improved survival rates can be expected only with early, accurate and reliable diagnosis followed by prompt and appropriate surgery. It seems that transvaginal color and pulsed Doppler could offer some improvements in the preoperative diagnosis of this rare disease. Chapter 2, devoted to the histopathology of the Fallopian tube, contains additional information on different tumors of this structure.

DIAGNOSIS OF PRIMARY FALLOPIAN TUBE CARCINOMA

In reviewing recent literature, several diagnostic methods have been found. Hysterosalpingography, laparoscopy and culdoscopy have all been utilized as aids to the clinical diagnosis of tubal carcinoma[6,18].

Hysterosalpingography is controversial, because of the possibility of spreading the cancer cells into the abdominal cavity when the contrast medium is injected into the tube, and therefore this procedure has almost been abandoned.

Exfoliative cytology had been suggested as a diagnostic tool when malignant glandular cells were present in vaginal smear with negative findings at the endometrial curettage[19–21]. It is important to note that no one has yet found cytologic features to distinguish cancers of tubal origin from cancers of the endometrium, the endocervix, or the ovary. Podobnik and colleagues[22] described the cells to be similar to an endometrioid-type ovarian carcinoma. If adenocarcinoma cells are found in the lower genital tract and there is no associated diathesis, an extrauterine source must be considered.

An antigen, present in most epithelial ovarian carcinomas as well as in other celomic epithelial neoplasms, such as the Fallopian tube epithelium, namely CA-125, has been reported recently as an important aid to the diagnosis of tubal carcinoma[23].

Table 1 B-mode diagnosis of Fallopian tube carcinoma

Reference	Number of cases	Findings	Histology
Subramayon et al. (1984)[26]	3	solid or cystic adnexal mass and sausage-like cystic masses with papillary projections	papillary cystadenocarcinoma
Ajjimakorn et al. (1988, 1991)[24, 25]	4	sausage-shaped cystic mass with papillary projections 5.3 × 2.1 cm	papillary cystadenocarcinoma
Meyer et al. (1987)[27]	1	sausage-shaped cystic mass with papillary projections 5.3 × 2.1 cm	adenocarcinoma
Granberg and Jannson (1990)[31]	1	left adnexal mass 4.2 × 2.4 cm	adenocarcinoma
Kol et al. (1990)[23]	1		
Chang et al. (1991)[11]	1	left adnexal mass 5 cm	adenocarcinoma and sarcoma (mixed Müllerian tumor)
Chiou et al. (1991)[10]	1		mixed Müllerian tumor

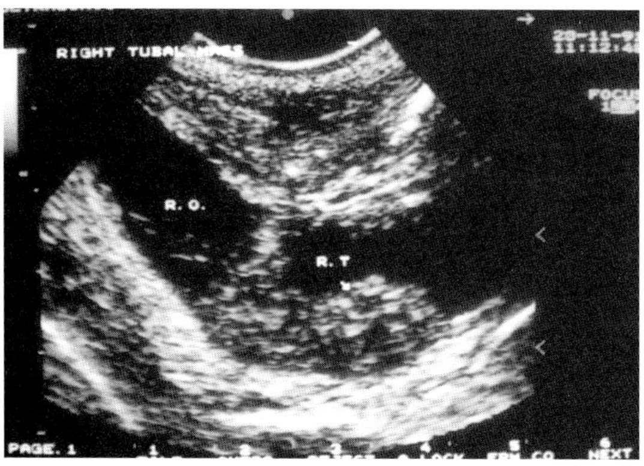

Figure 3 The complex right tubal mass (30×25 mm) is seen separate from the ipsilateral ovary (B-mode transvaginal sonography)

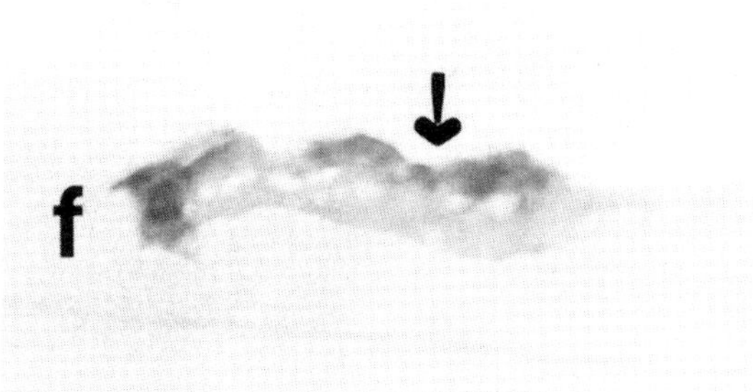

Figure 4 The right tubal mass (arrow) was incised to show the solid part of the mass; note that the serosa is not involved; f, fimbrial end of the tube

B-mode ultrasound

There are several publications on the successful preoperative diagnosis of Fallopian tube cancer by B-mode sonography[23-28]. Their results are analyzed and shown in Table 1. A tumor presented either as a cystic adnexal mass with internal papillary projections, or as an adnexal mass with mixed echogenicity with the normal-size ipsilateral ovary adjacent to the mass. Obviously, B-mode ultrasound can diagnose a tubal mass but cannot depict its exact nature accurately and reliably.

A significant diagnostic advance has been made by the introduction of transvaginal color and pulsed Doppler in the characterization of female pelvic tumors. Our group was the first to publish a case of primary adenocarcinoma of the Fallopian tube (stage I FIGO) in which color Doppler studies were helpful in arriving at the correct diagnosis[29]. This case and others are presented in detail below.

Case histories

A 50-year-old woman (gravida 2, para 1) presented with lower abdominal pain and vaginal discharge and was referred to the hospital after palpating an adnexal mass. Transvaginal B-mode (gray-scale) sonographic examination revealed a sausage-shaped cystic mass 30×25 mm, with solid parts (Figure 3). The mass was separate from the uterus as well as from the ipsilateral ovary. Transvaginal

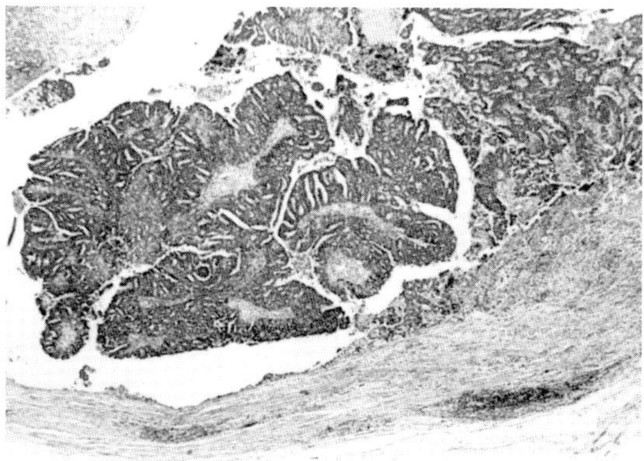

Figure 5 Tubal adenocarcinoma with intraluminal tumor growth, which does not infiltrate the wall of the tube

color Doppler sonography was carried out using the technique described in previous reports[30]. This revealed a 'hot' area which was evident within the solid part of the tumor. A RI of 0.35 and peak systolic velocity of 16.7 cm/s were measured (Color plates 16 and 17).

The diagnosis of tubal cancer was suspected on the basis of clinical and sonographic evaluations, namely, areas of neovascularization depicted by the color-rich area, and by the low RI detected by Doppler waveform analysis.

At laparotomy, a sausage-shaped complex mass involving the right tube was found (Figure 4). The other tube, both ovaries and the uterus were grossly normal. A tubal cancer stage I (FIGO classification) was diagnosed. Total abdominal hysterectomy and bilateral salpingo-oophorectomy were carried out. The histological diagnosis

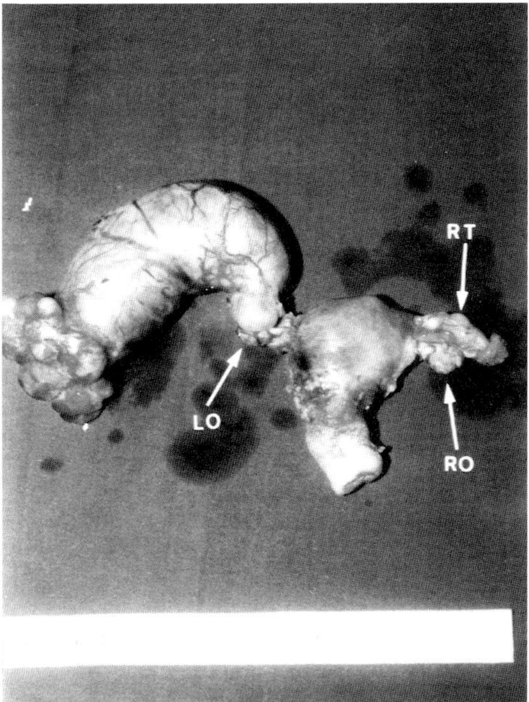

Figure 6 Primary carcinoma of the Fallopian tube. Pathological specimen showing a large left Fallopian tube measuring $14 \times 6 \times 4.5$ cm of fusiform appearance. The uterus, left ovary (LO), right ovary (RO) and the right tube (RT) were normal

confirmed the preoperative diagnosis of a papillary adenocarcinoma of the right tube, not infiltrating the tube wall (Figure 5). The left tube, both ovaries and the uterus were free of tumor cells.

More recently, we diagnosed another case of Fallopian tube carcinoma in a 52-year-old postmenopausal woman. The case is illustrated in Color plates 18 and 19.

A group from Valencia had another successful preoperative diagnosis. A 60-year-old woman, gravida 5, para 4, presented with postmenopausal bleeding and vaginal discharge which had persisted for the past 5 months. No abdominal pain was present. Pelvic examination revealed a palpable mass in the right adnexa. The Papanicolaou smear was read as normal (Type II). Transvaginal ultrasound revealed a $14 \times 6 \times 4$ cm sausage-shaped cystic mass, separated from the uterine fundus. This mass showed papillary projections extending from its inner surface (Color plate 20). The left adnexal mass was sepa-

rated from the uterus as well as the left ovary. Color Doppler studies demonstrated neovascularization within the solid part with an RI of 0.39 and a PI of 0.45. Fallopian tube carcinoma was suspected. Endometrial curettage was performed to rule out endometrial carcinoma, revealing an atrophic endometrium with no malignant lesions. At laparotomy, a large sausage-shaped complex mass involving the left tube was found. The right tube, both ovaries and the uterus were normal (Figure 6). Peritoneal washings were negative. Total abdominal hysterectomy with bilateral salpingo-oophorectomy, omentectomy and para-aortic and pelvic lymph node sampling were carried out. The surgical specimen showed a left Fallopian tube, measuring $14 \times 6 \times 4.5$ cm, of fusiform appearance. Upon sectioning, a grayish neoplastic growth, with necrotic and hemorrhagic areas, filled the lumen of the whole tube including the fimbriae, and apparently extended through the wall, but not beyond the serosal surface. The uterus seemed to be uninvolved with the tumor, presenting sessile polypoid endometrial areas, an intramural leiomyoma 1 cm in diameter, and a fibrous endocervix with small cysts. No lesions were found in the contralateral Fallopian tube. At the microscopic level, an epithelial neoplastic proliferation was found, showing papillary, glandular and solid (medullary) components, the latter with a marked nuclear pleomorphism and a high mitotic rate. Papillary areas with well-defined fibrovascular cores represented less than 25% of the tumor, and were of lower grade (Figure 7). Multiple foci of tumor necrosis were found with no association to any specific histologic pattern. In proximal and distal areas, the tumor was seen in continuity with normal, atrophic tubal epithelium (Figure 8). A thick, fibrous serosa covered the external surface of the tumor. The uterine corpus showed an atrophic endometrium, with prominent cystic change, giving a pseudopolypoid appearance. No neoplastic areas were found outside the left tube. A tubal primary carcinoma stage Ia (FIGO classification) was established.

Podobnik and co-workers[22] published the case of a 69-year-old woman, gravida 0, with a history of right-sided lower abdominal pain accompanied by profuse watery vaginal discharge for the past 3 months. Her general physical examination was normal. Inspection of the vulva, vagina and cervix

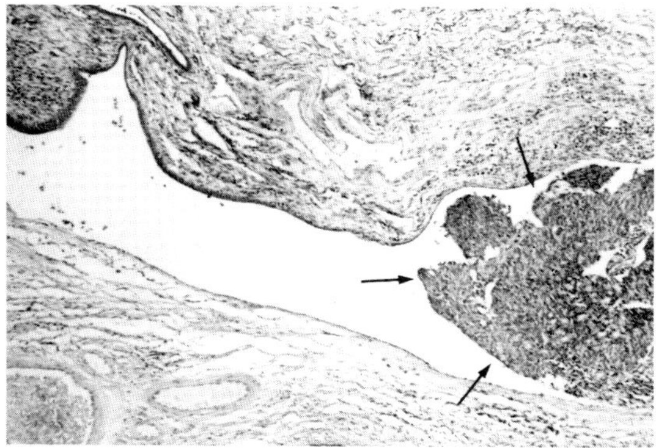

Figure 7 Microphotograph of the specimen in Figure 6. A solid, medullary pattern can be seen, showing pleomorphic tumor cells and several mitotic figures (arrows); H&E × 100

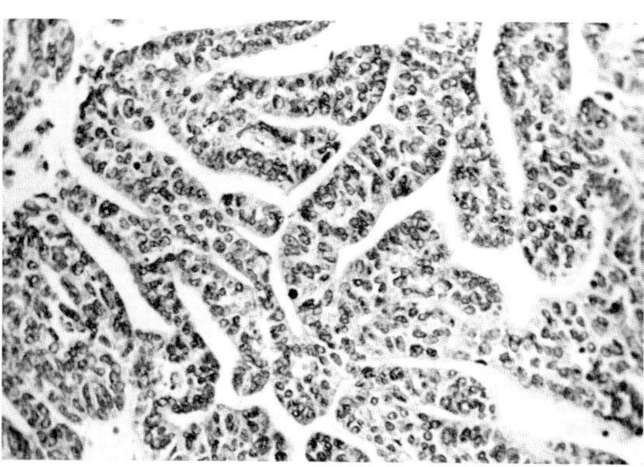

Figure 8 A well-defined papillary component of the tumor shown in Figures 6 and 7. Notice the fibrovascular cores as well as necrotic areas; H&E × 150

was unremarkable. No abnormal pelvic mass was palpable, but right adnexal fullness was suspected. The smear, which was a combined vaginal pool, cervical scrape and endocervical brush sample was generally 'clean' with no diathesis. In the vaginal pool, there was clean background, intermediary and basal vaginal squamous cells, and a few tumor cells in papillary clusters. Malignant cells were of moderate size, consistent with adenocarcinoma. Transvaginal sonography, using a 5-MHz transducer, demonstrated a right sausage-shaped cystic mass, size 6 × 4 × 2.5 cm, with papillary projections extending from the inner surface of the mass. The right ovary was small, size 2 × 2 cm, with normal

shape and echogenicity. During transvaginal examination, this mass changed in shape and size, accompanied by passage of free fluid through the uterine cavity. Superimposing color Doppler, a color-coded flow area was found at the periphery of the papillary structure of the right Fallopian tube. The PI was 0.62, and the RI was 0.34. Transvaginal color Doppler showed normal blood flow of the right ovary.

This ultrasonographic finding combined with the clinical presentation was highly suspicious of tubal malignancy. This suspicion was confirmed at surgery. Hysterectomy, bilateral salpingo-oophorectomy, appendectomy, partial omentectomy

Table 2 Fallopian tube carcinoma – transvaginal color Doppler diagnosis

Reference	Morphology	RI	Histology
Shalan and Kurjak (1992)[2]	sausage-shaped complex mass 3.0 × 2.5 cm with papillary projections	0.35	adenocarcinoma
Podobnik et al. (1993)[22]	sausage-shaped cystic mass 6.0 × 4.0 cm with papillary projections	0.34	clear-cell carcinoma
Bonilla-Musoles et al. (unpublished)	sausage-shaped cystic mass with papillary projections 14.0 × 6.0 cm	0.39	adenocarcinoma
Kurjak and Kupešić (unpublished)	sausage-shaped cystic mass with papillary projections	0.38	adenocarcinoma

RI, resistance index

and para-aortic and pelvic lymph node sampling were carried out. The histological diagnosis was clear cell carcinoma of the Fallopian tube with a normal right ovary. Serum assay of CA-125 a few days after surgery indicated a level of 20 U/ml.

All four illustrated cases displayed tumor neovascularization which was detectable by color Doppler imaging (Table 2). They all had resistance indices below 0.40. These promising findings demonstrate the potential of transvaginal color Doppler to depict this rare tubal cancer, and to bring it to early treatment.

References

1. Woodruff, J.D. and Pauerstein, C.J. (1969). *The Fallopian Tube.* (Baltimore: Williams and Wilkins)
2. Mroueh, J., Margono, F. and Feinkind, L. (1993). Tubal pregnancy associated with ampullary tubal leiomyoma. *Obstet. Gynecol.*, **81**, 880–2
3. Timor-Tritsch, I.E. and Rottem, S. (1987). Transvaginal ultrasonographic study of the Fallopian tube. *Obstet. Gynecol.*, **70**, 424–8
4. McGoldrick, J.L., Strauss, H. and Rao, J. (1943). Primary carcinoma of the Fallopian tube. *Am. J. Surg.*, **59**, 559–63
5. Eddy, G.L., Schlaerth, J.B., Nalick, R.H., Gadis, O.J., Nakmura, R.M. and Morrow, C.P. (1984). Fallopian tube carcinoma. *Obstet. Gynecol.*, **64**, 546–51
6. Podratz, K.C., Schray, M.F., Rock, M., Martinez, A. and Howes, A.E. (1986). Primary carcinoma of the Fallopian tube. *Am. J. Obstet. Gynecol.*, **154**, 1319–26
7. Ayhan, A., Deren, D., Yuce, K., Tuncer, Z. and Mecan, G. (1994). Primary carcinoma of the Fallopian tube: a study of 8 cases. *Eur. J. Gynecol. Oncol.*, **15**, 147–51
8. Dava, D., Young, R.H. and Scully, R.E. (1992). Endometrioid carcinoma of the Fallopian tube resembling an adnexal tumor of probable Wolffian origin: a report of six cases. *Int. J. Gynecol. Pathol.*, **11**, 122–30
9. Soundara, R.S., Ramdas, C.P., Reddi, R.P., Oumachigni, A., Rajaram, P. and Reddy, K.S. (1991). A review of Fallopian tube carcinoma over 20 years (1971–90) in Pondicherry. *Indian J. Cancer*, **28**, 188–95
10. Chiou, Y.K., Su, I.J., Chen, C.A. and Hsieh, C.Y. (1991). Malignant mixed Müllerian tumor of the Fallopian tube. *J. Formos. Med. Assoc.*, **90**, 793–5
11. Chang, H.C., Hsueh, S. and Soong, Y.K. (1991). Malignant mixed Müllerian tumor of the Fallopian tube. Case report and review of literature. *Chang Keng I Hsueh Med. J.*, **14**, 259–63
12. Tokunaga, T., Miyazaki, K. and Okamura, H. (1991). Pathology of the Fallopian tube. *Curr. Opin. Obstet. Gynecol.*, **3**, 574–9
13. Rosen, A., Klein, M., Lahousen, M., Graf, A.H., Rainer, A. and Vavra, N. (1993). Primary carcinoma of the Fallopian tube – retrospective analysis of 115 patients. *Br. J. Cancer*, **68**, 605–9
14. Hu, C.Y. and Cheng, F.K. (1959). Histological findings of the tubal malignancies. *Chin. Med. J.*, **76**, 517–28
15. Roberts, J.A. and Lifshitz, S. (1982). Primary adenocarcinoma of the Fallopian tube. *Gynecol. Oncol.*, **13**, 301–7
16. Sedlis, A. (1978). Carcinoma of the Fallopian tube. *Surg. Clin. North. Am.*, **58**, 121–6
17. Jacoby, A.F., Fuller, A.R., Thor, A.D. and Muntz, H.G. (1993). Primary leiomyosarcoma of the Fallopian tube. *Gynecol. Oncol.*, **51**, 404–7
18. Engstrom, L. (1957). Primary carcinoma of the Fallopian tube. *Acta Obstet. Gynecol. Scand.*, **36**, 289–305
19. Sedlis, A. (1961). Primary carcinoma of the Fallopian tube. *Obstet. Gynecol. Surv.*, **16**, 209–226
20. Larsson, E. and Schooley, J.L. (1960). Positive vaginal cytology in primary tubal carcinoma. *Am. J. Obstet. Gynecol.*, **72**, 1364–6
21. Schenck, S.B. and Mackles, A. (1961). Primary carcinoma of the Fallopian tubes with positive smears. *Am. J. Obstet. Gynecol.*, **81**, 782–3
22. Podobnik, M., Singer, Z., Ciglar, S. and Bulić, M. (1993). Preoperative diagnosis of primary Fallopian tube carcinoma by transvaginal ultrasound, cytological finding and CA-125. *Ultrasound Med. Biol.*, **19**, 587–91
23. Kol, S., Gal, D., Friedman, M. and Paldi, E. (1990). Preoperative diagnosis of Fallopian tube carcinoma by transvaginal sonography and CA-125. *Gynecol. Oncol.*, **37**, 129–31
24. Ajjimakorn, S., Bhamarapravati, Y. and Israngura, N. (1988). Ultrasound appearance of Fallopian tube carcinoma (case report). *J. Clin. Ultrasound*, **16**, 516–18
25. Ajjimakorn, S. and Bhamarapravati, Y. (1991). Transvaginal ultrasound and the diagnosis of Fallopian tubal carcinoma. *J. Clin. Ultrasound*, **19**, 116–19
26. Subramayon, B.R., Raghavendra, B.N., Whalen, C.A. and Yee, J. (1984). Ultrasonic features of Fallopian tube carcinoma. *J. Ultrasound Med.*, **3**, 391–3
27. Meyer, J.S., Kim, C.S., Price, H.M. and Cooke, J.K.

(1987). Ultrasound presentation of primary carcinoma of the Fallopian tube. *J. Clin. Ultrasound*, **15**, 132–4

28. Hinton, A., Bea, C., Winfield, A.C. and Entman, S.S. (1988). Carcinoma of the Fallopian tube. *Krol. Radiol.*, **10**, 113–15

29. Shalan, H., Sosic, A. and Kurjak, A. (1992). Fallopian tube carcinoma: recent diagnostic approach by color Doppler imaging. *Ultrasound Obstet. Gynecol.*, **2**, 297–9

30. Kurjak, A., Zalud, I., Jurkovic, D., Alfirevic, Z. and Miljan, M. (1989). Transvaginal color Doppler for the assessment of pelvic circulation. *Acta Obstet. Gynecol. Scand.*, **68**, 131–5

31. Granberg, S. and Jansson, I. (1990). Early detection of primary carcinoma of the Fallopian tube by endovaginal ultrasound. *Acta Obstet. Gynecol. Scand.*, **69**, 667–8.

Paratubal tumors: sonographic appearance

9

N. Haratz-Rubinstein, I. E. Timor-Tritsch and A. Monteagudo

INTRODUCTION

When the adnexa are scanned, structures can appear clearly belonging to the ovary, the Fallopian tube or the vessels around it or to the cul-de-sac and its lateral extensions. However, all those who make imaging their main interest know that in many instances a structure cannot be accurately traced back to the ovary or the Fallopian tube due to its bizarre non-diagnostic shape or location. At other times, embryological remnants give rise to structures not usually present in the pelvis, making them more difficult to diagnose correctly.

This short chapter deals with relatively rare and interesting sonographic findings in the adnexal area. They may be important as the differential diagnostic process is followed in the case of adnexal sonography.

BACKGROUND

Paraovarian or paratubal tumors are those which are located in the broad ligament but are completely separated from and not connected with either the ovary or the uterus[1]. They are mostly cystic structures but solid and complex masses have also been described[1,2]. From a sonographic point of view, the more relevant are the cystic paraovarian tumors because of their higher frequency and the greater size that they may attain[2,3].

Paraovarian cysts can be divided according to their embryological origin into three main categories[4]:

(1) Mesothelial: peritoneal inclusion cysts;

(2) Paramesonephric: hydatid cyst of Morgagni; and

(3) Mesonephric: Kobelt's cyst, cysts of the paraoophoron and cysts of the rete ovarii.

In order to avoid further confusion and for practical purposes, only the names of the three main categories will be used. Other conditions that have been less frequently found in the broad ligaments include: lymphocysts, Walthard cell rests, heterotopic adrenal cortical rests, endosalpingiosis, endometriosis, nodular fasciitis (pseudosarcomatous fasciitis), Mülleroma and pelvic hydatid cysts[4]. A detailed description of these structures is beyond the scope of this chapter.

To understand better the pathological basis of paraovarian cysts, a brief review of the embryology of the female genital ducts is warranted. Both male and female embryos have two pairs of genital or sex ducts. The mesonephric or Wolffian ducts play an important role in the development of the male reproductive system, and the paramesonephric or Müllerian ducts play an important role in the development of the female reproductive system[5].

In female embryos, the mesonephric ducts mostly regress but at least the caudal one-third and some 10–15 mesonephric tubules connected to the cranial part are consistently preserved and persists as such throughout adult life[1]. The paramesonephric ducts develop into the Fallopian tubes, uterus and the superior part of the vagina. As the Fallopian tubes develop, occasional accessory tubules of paramesonephric origin may form due to the compression of their terminal ends between the receding pronephros and the mesonephric body[6]. These miniature tubes may be attached to the broad ligament anywhere.

The mesonephric and paramesonephric derivatives previously described are normal structures of the adult broad ligament. They may distend, developing into the so-called paraovarian cysts which are not true tumors, but merely distension phenomena. Their walls are composed of thin compressed connective tissue and muscle fibers in contrast to true neoplasms in which the fibrous tissue wall takes an active part in tumor growth[1]. Paraovarian cysts can also arise from the mesothelium that covers the adnexal peritoneum (peritoneal inclusion cysts).

The majority of paraovarian cysts are of para-mesonephric or mesothelial origin[3,5,7,8]. Genadry and colleagues[2] found that, of 132 paraovarian cysts, 67% were of mesothelial origin, 31% para-mesonephric and 2% mesonephric. On the other hand, Samaha and co-workers[6] reported that 76% of 79 paratubal cysts were of paramesonephric origin.

Paraovarian cysts commonly occur in the fourth and fifth decades of life[3], with a range between 10 and 79 years[2]. Reported symptoms include pelvic pain, menstrual disorder and pelvic 'heaviness'[3]. Complications include torsion of the cyst or even of the whole adnexa, due to the fact that these masses can act as a fulcrum to potentiate the torsion of the ovary and Fallopian tube[9]. Malignant degeneration has also been described with a low incidence of 5.71%[2], 75% of them being papillary serous cystadenocarcinomas. Other reported complications are hemorrhage, rupture and secondary infection[8].

Gynecological pathologies that have been reported in patients with paraovarian tumors are uterine fibromyomas, uterine prolapse and ovarian and cervical cancer. Also, paraovarian cysts can modify normal tubal anatomy, thus affecting zygote transfer and predisposing to ectopic pregnancy[3].

Case report

A 15-year-old adolescent, gravida 0, was seen in the emergency room complaining of sudden onset right lower quadrant pain and vomiting for 3 hours prior to admission. She denied fever, diarrhea, or urinary symptoms. Her last menstrual period was 3 weeks prior to presentation. She was sexually active. There was no prior medical or surgical history.

On admission, the patient was calm, blood pressure 90/60 mmHg, pulse 80 beats/min,

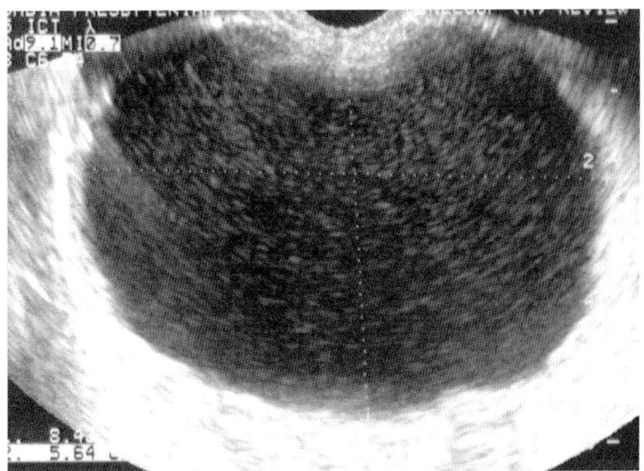

Figure 1 Transvaginal sonographic picture of a cystic structure in the right adnexa showing low-level echoes. The pathology report was consistent with a paratubal cyst with hemorrhagic infarction

respiratory rate 20 and temperature 98 F. Cardiopulmonary examination was unremarkable. The abdomen showed bowel sounds; it was soft, with mild lower quadrant and flank tenderness. There was no rebound or guarding. Gynecological examination revealed normal external genitalia with no vaginal discharge. The uterus was anteverted, 8 weeks size, globular non-tender. A right non-tender adnexal mass was noted. The left adnexa was normal to palpation. Her white count was 11 000/mm[3], hematocrit 32.3%; urine analysis and pregnancy tests were negative.

A transabdominal and transvaginal sonographic evaluation performed 24 hours before laparotomy revealed an axial uterus measuring 7.9 × 3.9 cm with an endometrial width of 1.26 cm. The left ovary contained several small follicles and measured 3.4 × 1.9 cm. In the midline, just on top of the uterus and pushing it posteriorly, there was a cystic mass 8.4 × 5.6 cm with low-level echoes within (Figure 1). On the right adnexa a 5.35 × 4.01 cm complex mass was noted, containing several cystic structures mainly in the center. No flow was demonstrated by color Doppler. There was fluid in the cul-de-sac and surrounding the right adnexa.

An exploratory laparotomy revealed a dilated right adnexa measuring approximately 7 cm. It appeared multiloculated and was torsed three times around the pedicle. The right ovary was enlarged, measuring approximately 6 cm. A right salpingo-oophorectomy and appendectomy were

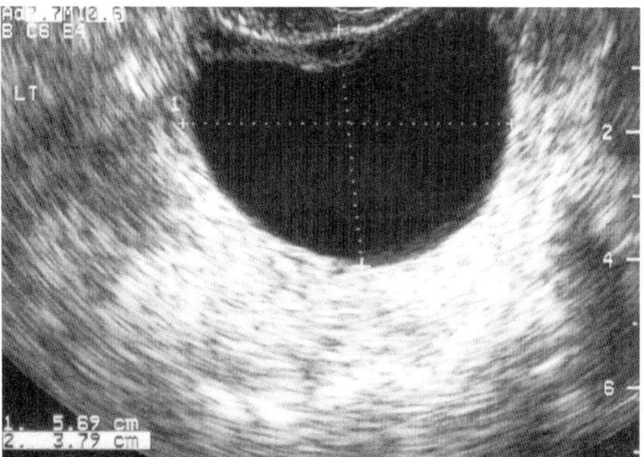

Figure 2 Adnexa showing a sonolucent paraovarian cyst with a thin smooth wall

performed. The postoperative course was unremarkable. The pathological findings were consistent with a paratubal cyst and ovary with hemorrhagic infection.

SONOGRAPHIC ASPECTS

Paraovarian cysts represent one of the sonographic differential diagnoses of adnexal masses.

Usually they are unilocular sonolucent structures with smooth, thin walls (Figure 2), that may be identical to simple follicular cysts, but they arise from the adnexa rather than the ovary (Figure 3)[10]. A curious feature of paraovarian cysts, present in the aforementioned case report, is their frequent location superior to the uterus. Athey and Cooper[11], in a series of eight paraovarian cysts, reported six to be in this location. They suggested, that as paraovarian cysts enlarge, they may migrate out of the pelvis due to the mobility conferred by the broad ligament.

Pepe and colleagues[3] found 86% of 59 cases to be unilateral, with no predominance of either side. In their series, 49% were between 6 and 10 cm in dimension, although they can attain larger sizes. Hutchinson reported a paraovarian cyst containing 36 000 ml of fluid[12]. Cysts over 5 cm are customary in the younger population and most of these larger cysts have been found to be of the mesothelial variety. Logically, they are the most symptomatic, necessitating surgical intervention[2].

The hydatid or cyst of Morgagni is the most common paramesonephric cyst. They are usually found dangling from one end of the fimbriae and can measure up to 10 mm[8], although larger masses

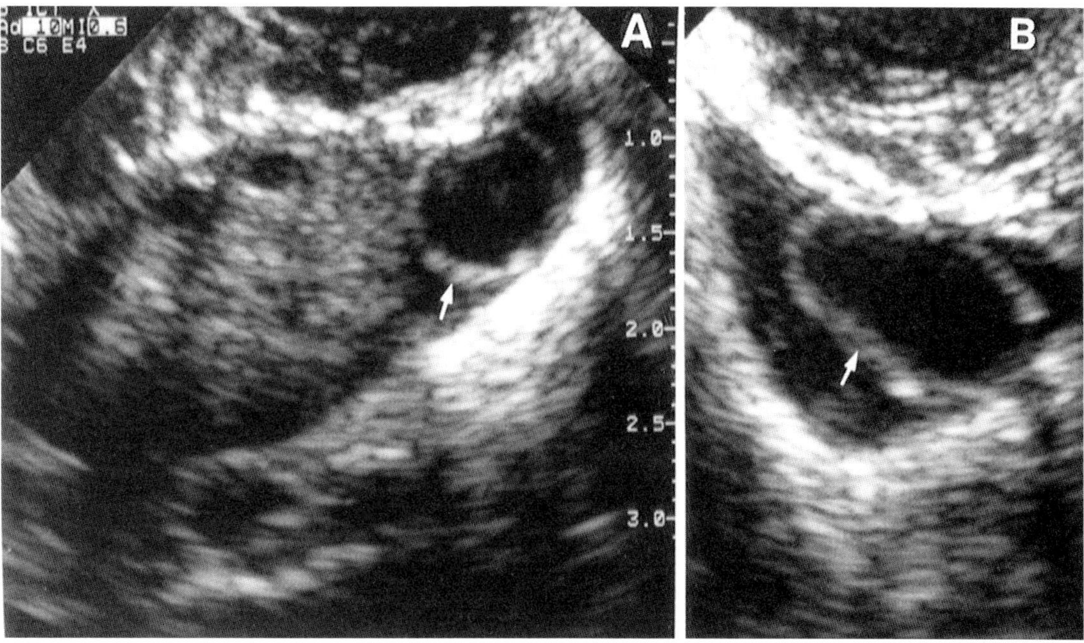

Figure 3 Transvaginal view of the adnexa. A, The ovary can be seen separated from a round sonolucent structure (arrow); B, in the same patient the arrow points to a longitudinal view of the sonolucent structure depicted in A. The pathology report was consistent with a hydatid cyst of Morgagni

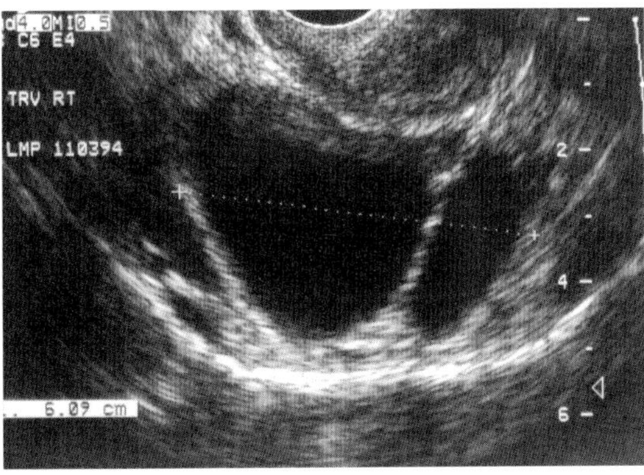

Figure 4 Peritoneal inclusion cyst. Transvaginal scan shows a multiloculated cyst with sonolucent areas and thin septa. Sonolucent areas represent fluid trapped between pelvic adhesions. Differential diagnosis with an ovarian neoplasm depends on its visualization as a separated structure

measuring up to 30 mm have been found (personal experience).

Paraovarian cysts of mesothelial origin have been designated as peritoneal inclusion cysts, pseudocysts[10], or less frequently as benign cystic mesotheliomas[13]. These lesions can vary from unilocular cysts measuring 7–10 cm to multilocular cysts measuring up to 15 cm. They are characterized by walls and septa composed of inflamed fibrous, granulation tissue and mesothelial cells with no involvement of the substance of the ipsilateral ovary or tube (Figure 4). It has been theorized that fluid that is normally produced by the ovaries is trapped in the pelvis by peritoneal adhesions, forming these so-called peritoneal inclusion cysts. In addition, the inflammatory process that is frequently observed in these peritoneal adhesions may decrease the normal clearance of ovarian fluid and may by itself cause an exudate. In these patients, peritoneal adhesions may be the result of prior abdominal surgery, pelvic inflammatory disease, or endometriosis[14]. The diagnosis of paraovarian cyst of mesothelial origin (peritoneal inclusion cyst) should be considered when a patient with such a history presents with a pelvic multiloculated mass on sonographic evaluation.

Differential diagnosis of paraovarian cysts with ovarian neoplasms can be difficult unless the ipsilateral ovary can be demonstrated sonographically to be separated from the cyst (Figure 5).

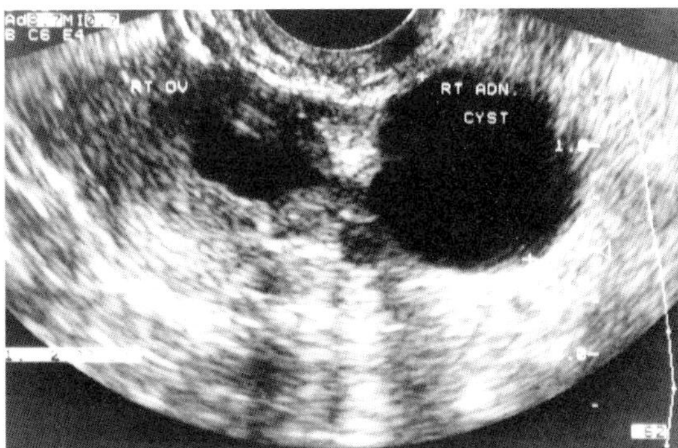

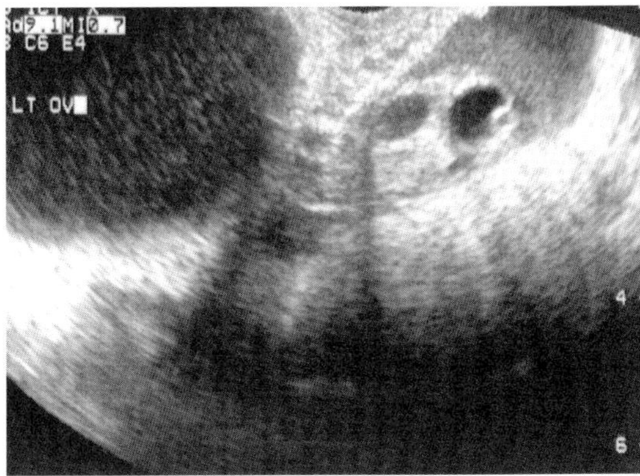

Figure 5 Transvaginal sonographic picture of the adnexa showing the ovary separated from a cystic sonolucent structure. This is the most important differential diagnostic feature of a paraovarian cyst. Top, A paraovarian cyst in the right adnexa; bottom, left adnexa showing a simple sonolucent structure with low-level echoes. To the right a normal ovary can be seen separated and surrounded by fluid

Unfortunately, this ovary is seldom seen due to the marked adnexal distortion caused by the paraovarian cyst resulting in displacement and obscuration with bowel or fat[11]. The fact that ovarian physiologic cysts can be expected to change in size over the menstrual cycle and with the administration of hormonal compounds such as contraceptive pills can help to distinguish them from paraovarian cysts, with maybe the exception of peritoneal inclusion cysts. These, being filled at least in part with fluid of ovarian origin, can also be expected to change in the above-mentioned situations.

Paraovarian cysts can also resemble endometriomas, specially if they are hemorrhagic (Figure 1), with the difference that endometriomas tend to have a more irregular wall[15]. Teratomas would be more complex structures, commonly presenting with highly echogenic foci with acoustic shadowing representing calcification from teeth or other elements.

A hydrosalpinx could occasionally be indistinguishable from a paraovarian cyst, although dilated Fallopian tubes can usually be characterized by tubular shape, folded configuration and short linear echoes protruding into the lumen[16]. In the case of a tubo-ovarian abscess, the most common sonographic appearance is a complex, hypoechoic adnexal mass with variable septations, irregular margins, scattered internal echoes and fluid debris levels[17]. Also, the clinical manifestations of pelvic inflammatory disease would help in making the correct diagnosis.

Almost any type of ovarian tumor can occur in the broad ligament, perhaps arising in accessory ovarian tissue[18] and developing into solid paraovarian masses with similar sonographic features as their ovarian counterparts. In this setting, differential diagnosis between ovarian or paraovarian would seem hardly possible unless, as previously mentioned, the ipsilateral ovary could be separately visualized. Transvaginal sonography, through its higher frequency and resolution, can be of invaluable help in identifying the ovaries, thus narrowing the diagnostic possibilities.

A wide variety of benign and malignant broad ligament tumors of less clinical relevance has been described in the literature[1, 7, 18–20], including epithelial as well as mesenchymal neoplasms. They are commonly solid strucutres, with more pathologic than sonographic interest. Among them are leiomyomas, fibromas, lipomas, papillary serous cystadenoma and cystadenofibromas, extra-ovarian Brenner tumors, thecomas, heterotopic adrenal cell adenomas and granulosa cell tumors.

Malignant primary tumors of the broad ligament include sarcomas, adenocarcinomas of probable paramesonephric origin and mesonephric carcinomas. Metastases to the broad ligament are also possible. Three categories have been described:

(1) Superficial spread of tumor along the serosa (ovarian carcinoma);

(2) Metastases located between the leaflets of the broad ligament (endometrial, cervical, rectosigmoid and urinary bladder carcinomas); and

(3) Metastases to the lymph nodes located in the broad ligament (cervical carcinomas).

Lymphomas and leukemias may also involve the broad ligaments secondarily[20]. These malignant tumors of the broad ligament should be considered as a differential diagnosis when an adnexal complex mass separated from the ovary is detected by ultrasound in a postmenopausal woman.

References

1. Gardner, G.H., Green, R.R. and Peckam, B. (1957). Tumors of the broad ligament. *Am. J. Obstet. Gynecol.*, **73**, 536–54

2. Genadry, R., Parmley, T. and Woodruff, J.D. (1977). The origin and clinical behavior of the paraovarian tumor. *Am. J. Obstet. Gynecol.*, **129**, 873–9

3. Pepe, F., Panella, M., Pepe, G. and Panella, P. (1986). Paraovarian tumors. *Eur. J. Gynaecol. Oncol.*, **8**, 159–60

4. Janovsky, N.A. and Paramanandhan, T.L. (1973). Tumorous conditions of the Fallopian tubes and ligaments of the female reproductive organs. In Janovsky, N.A. and Paramanandhan, T.L. (eds.) *Ovarian Tumors: Tumors and Tumor like Conditions of the Ovaries, Fallopian Tubes, and Ligaments of the Uterus*, pp. 191–203. (Philadelphia: W.B. Saunders)

5. Moore, K.L. (1988). The urogenital system. In Moore, K.L. (ed.) *The Developing Human*, pp. 267–8.

(Philadelphia: W.B. Saunders)

6. Samaha, M. and Woodruff, J.D. (1985). Paratubal cysts: frequency, histogenesis and associated clinical features. *Obstet. Gynecol.*, **65**, 691–3

7. Wheeler, J.E. (1987). Diseases of the Fallopian tube. In Kurman, R.J. (ed.) *Blaunstein's Pathology of the Female Genital Tract*, 3rd edn., pp. 430–2. (New York: Springer-Verlag)

8. Alpern, M.B., Sandler, M.A. and Madrazo, B.L. (1984). Sonographic features of paraovarian cysts and their complications. *Am. J. Roentgenol.*, **143**, 157–60

9. Graif, M. and Itzhack, Y. (1988). Sonographic evaluation of ovarian torsion in childhood and adolescence. *Am. J. Roentgenol.*, **150**, 647–9

10. Grant, E.G. (1992). Benign conditions of the ovaries. In Nyberg, D.A., Hill, L.M., Bohm-Velez, M. and Mendelson, E.B. (eds.) *Transvaginal Ultrasound,*

pp. 197–208. (St. Louis, Missouri. Mosby Year-book)

11. Athey, P.A. and Cooper, N.B. (1985). Sonographic features of paraovarian cysts. *Am. J. Roentgenol.*, **144**, 83–6

12. Hutchinson, M.E. (1939). Intraligamentous paraovarian cyst. *Am. J. Obstet. Gynecol.*, **37**, 505–6

13. McFadden, D.E. and Clement, P.B. (1986). Peritoneal inclusion cysts with mural mesothelial proliferation. *Am. J. Surg. Pathol.*, **10**, 844–54

14. Hoffer, F.A., Kozakewich, H., Colodny, A. and Goldstein, D.P. (1988). Peritoneal inclusion cysts: ovarian fluid in peritoneal adhesions. *Radiology*, **169**, 189–91

15. Sandler, M.A., Silver, T.M. and Karo, J.J. (1978). The spectrum of ultrasonic findings in endometriosis. *Radiology*, **127**, 229–31

16. Tessler, F.N., Perrella, R.R., Fleischer, A.C. and Grant, E.G. (1989). Endovaginal sonographic diagnosis of dilated Fallopian tubes. *Am. J. Roentgenol.*, **153**, 523–5

17. Patten, R.M. (1992). The Fallopian tube and pelvic inflammatory disease. In Nyberg, D.A., Hill, I.M., Bohm-Velez, M. and Mendelson, E.B. (eds.) *Transvaginal Ultrasound*, pp. 215–21. (St. Louis, Missouri: Mosby Year-book)

18. Zaloudeck, C.H. (1994). The ovary. In Gompel, C. and Silverberg, S.G. (eds.) *Pathology in Gynecology and Obstetrics*, 4th edn., pp. 401–2. (Philadelphia: J.B. Lippincott)

19. Wild, R.A., Albert, R.D., Zaino, R.J. and Abrams, C.S. (1988). Virilizing paraovarian tumors: a consequence of Nelson's syndrome. *Obstet. Gynecol.*, **71**, 1053–6

20. Janovsky, N.A. and Paramanandhan, T.L. (1973). Tumors of the ligaments of the female reproductive organs. In Janovsky, N.A. and Paramanandhan, T.L. (eds.) *Ovarian Tumors: Tumors and Tumor like Conditions of the Ovaries, Fallopian Tubes and Ligaments of the Uterus*, pp. 182–90. (Philadelphia: W.B. Saunders)

Evaluation of tubal patency by color Doppler hysterosalpingography 10

S. Kupešić and A. Kurjak

The number of cases of tubal sterility is increasing and tubal factors, such as tubal dysfunction or obstruction, account for approximately 35% of the causes of infertility[1,2]. A history of pelvic inflammatory disease, septic abortion, intra-uterine contraceptive device use, ruptured appendix, tubal surgery, or ectopic pregnancy should alter the physician to the possibility of tubal damage. One aspect of the infertility investigation which has changed little over the last 20 years is that of the assessment of Fallopian tube patency. In 1954, Rubin[3] described the use of the first attempt to assess tubal patency. The diagnosis of tubal factor traditionally has been made by insufflating the Fallopian tubes. Until now, the most frequently used procedures to demonstrate tubal patency have been X-ray hysterosalpingo-graphy and chromopertubation during laparo-scopy[4].

Hysterosalpingography, using radio-opaque dye for X-ray studies to assess tubal and uterine anatomy, has been the standard form of investigation for several decades. The disadvantage of this type of investigation is that ionizing radiation has inherent risks to the oocyte, which may result in congenital malformations, if conception takes place in the investigatory cycle. Furthermore, known allergy to iodine-containing dyes is a contraindication to X-ray hysterosalpingography (Table 1).

Debate continues as to the most appropriate hysterosalpingography medium: oil - or water-based. Water-soluble medium flows more freely through the uterus, is rapidly absorbed and more of the medium is needed. It allows delineation of the rugal pattern of the ampulla and, therefore, provides prognostic information in cases of distal tubal obstruction. Oil-based medium does not mix with accumulated fluid in hydrosalpinges.

However, it has been associated (albeit only rarely) with granulomata formation in the pelvic tissues with oil emboli. Proponents claim that the oil-based medium incurs less pain and is able to delineate more sharply abnormalities in the uterine luminal contour. Furthermore, a higher pregnancy rate has been reported by some inves-tigators following hysterosalpingography with oil-based medium when compared to water-based[5].

Hysteroscopy is a technique which comple-ments hysterosalpingography. It can accurately differentiate between endometrial polyps and submucous leiomyomas, and can be used for their treatment. The same method is useful in estab-lishing the definitive diagnosis and treatment of intrauterine adhesions and some congenital anomalies of the uterus (Table 1).

Hysteroscopy-directed falloposcopy can detect obstruction of the tubal ostium, and can be utilized to examine the entire length of the tubal lumen[6]. Treatment of the proximal tubal obstruc-tion can immediately follow the diagnosis. Transcervical tubal cannulation or balloon tubo-plasty performed by hysteroscopic approach are the methods of choice[7]. It is hoped that further development of the modern technology will allow these interventions to be performed in outpatient clinics using ultrasonography.

Laparoscopy, to investigate tubal status, has been used as the gold standard in the last two decades, but this requires a general anesthetic and carries the risk of surgical complications, such as bowel or vascular injury[8], false pneumoperi-toneum and postoperative discomfort. With a Jarcho-type of cannula in the uterine cavity, one can manipulate the uterus, and, by instilling indigo–carmine saline, or other tinted saline, can test for tubal competence.

Table 1 Relative merits of laparoscopy, hysteroscopy, X-ray hysterosalpingography (HSG) and color Doppler hysterosalpingography used for obtaining information on tubal patency

	X-ray HSG	Hysteroscopy	Laparoscopy	Color Doppler HSG
Anesthesia	not required	+/- general	general	not required
Risks	pelvic inflammatory disease dye sensitivity infection	+/- anesthetic risks perforation hemorrhage infection	anesthetic risks intra-abdominal trauma hemorrhage infection	pelvic inflammatory disease infection
Facilities	X-ray machine fluoroscope	+/- operating room	operating room	color Doppler equipment
Benefits	opacification of tubal lumen (ampullary rugal pattern, intramural or intraluminal abnormalities of the Fallopian tube)	visualization of endometrial cavity (polyps, synechia, leiomyomas, septum and other anomalies) and tubal ostium allows immediate treatment	visualization of peritoneal surfaces (adhesions, pelvic organs, endometriosis) allows immediate treatment	avoidance of the ionization and idiosyncrasy to contrast media easily repeatable requires intraprocedural active participation of the patient (increases her knowledge of tubal status) is a dynamic procedure analyzing tubal motility the procedure course is stored, reviewed, analyzed and interpreted to the infertile couple using video-recorder the most illustrative photos (representing uterine cavity and tubal patency) are easily obtainable from the video material does not require equipment of the Radiology Department (decreasing of the cost)
Cost	+	++	+++	+

Through laparoscopy one is equally able to visualize the total pelvic anatomy and the upper abdominal cavity. It is also useful for evaluation of ovarian disease, genital anomalies, tubal and adnexal competence, and to differentiate between pelvic distortions. Furthermore, it is valuable to reach an accurate classification of endometriosis of the pelvis. Laparoscopy can be used as an adjunct in assessing possible causes of pelvic pain, the extent of pelvic neoplasia, as well as for a prognostic review of a previous infertility surgical procedure. It has also been helpful in obtaining peritoneal washings and cultures in patients with positive history of pelvic inflammatory disease (Table 1).

Ultrasound imaging of the pelvic organs has improved significantly with the use of high-frequency vaginal ultrasound probes where the need for bladder filling can be avoided. The normal Fallopian tube is usually not seen by vaginal sonography unless some fluid surrounds it. This contrasting fluid may be one of the following:

(1) The normal serous fluid present in the pelvis of a large number of healthy patients;

(2) Follicular fluid during or after ovulation;

(3) Blood;

(4) Ascitic fluid; or

(5) Products of an exudative or infectious process, namely, a purulent fluid.

If the Fallopian tube is not filled with fluid, its lumen cannot be detected[9].

Richman and colleagues[10] were the first to report on the transabdominal sonographic evaluation of tubal patency (Color plates 21 and 22). In their studies they used a special intrauterine catheter, Harris uterine injector (Unimar, Canoga Park, CA). After injection of at least 20 ml of the ultrasonic contrast medium Hyskon (dextron in dextrose; Pharmacia Laboratories, Piscataway, NJ), the accumulation of fluid in the cul-de-sac has been accepted as an indicator of tubal patency.

Randolph and co-workers[11] used transabdominal ultrasound for observation of the cul-de-sac after the injection of 200 ml isotonic saline through the Rubin cannula. The presence of retrouterine fluid was accepted as a criterion for patency of one or both tubes.

Tubal patency was deduced indirectly from the presence of increasing fluid in the pouch of Douglas, without differentiation of the sides.

A new transvaginal ultrasonographic technique was developed in 1989 by Deichert and colleagues[12]. They visualized the patent tube directly and hence showed tubal patency by transcervical injection of an echogenic and ultrasonic contrast fluid SHU 454 (Echovist; Schering, Berlin, Germany). The method has been called Hy-Co-Sy: transvaginal hysterosalpingo-contrast sonography. They used Rubin Cannula or a bladder catheter no. 8. The same researchers have continued their studies on transvaginal hystero-contrast sonography[10,13] under general anesthesia. Tüfekci and co-workers[14] have developed an easier technique in which the patient does not require hospitalization. By intrauterine injection of isotonic saline, they evaluated tubal patency directly and called this method transvaginal sonosalpingography.

Transvaginal sonosalpingography performed by using isotonic saline without anesthesia is physiological, easy to perform, safe, cost-effective, non-invasive and more convenient when compared with other conventional methods. Idiosyncrasy to the contrast agent cannot be expected.

All media having a different echogenicity from that of the human body can be used as contrast media. Contrast media are divided into two groups: hypoechogenic and hyperechogenic media.

Isotonic saline, Ringer or dextran solutions belong to the first group. Instillation of these media facilitates the detection of echogenic border surfaces. The main disadvantage is that it is not possible to visualize the phenomena of motion and flow.

Hyperechogenic contrast media enhance echo signals, allowing detection of the flow by both B-mode and Doppler ultrasound. Gramiak and Shah[15] and Meltzer and co-workers[16] found that small gas bubbles effectively reflect ultrasonic waves. Therefore, all the commercial echo contrast media contain microbubbles. Commercial products Echovist and Levovist (Schering AG, Berlin) represent suspension of microbubbles made of special galactose microparticles. Galactose microparticle granules are suspended either in galactose solution (Echovist) or in a sterile water (Levovist)[17]. After injection of this microbubble suspension containing galactose, cavities of blood become echogenic, until these microparticles have dissolved. Numerous clinical studies in the field of echocardiography, venous vascular system analysis and hysterosalpingography showed no evidence of serious side-effects. Absolute contraindication for instillation of these fluids is galactosemia (autosomal recessive disease in which, due to a deficiency of galactose-1-phosphate uridyltransferase, galactose cannot be metabolized into glucose).

Further advantages of transvaginal sonosalpingography include the possibility of performing the procedure on an outpatient basis. This has significantly altered the need for inpatient facilities at some infertility departments[18].

However, the information gained by both procedures is critically dependent on both the technical skill and experience of the operator, as well as on the proper interpretation. Bleeding, pregnancy, presence of adnexal masses on pelvic or ultrasound examination are contraindications to color Doppler hysterosalpingography.

Ultrasound examination prior to the procedure is necessary to define uterine position and anomalies if present (Color plate 23) as well as both adnexal regions. The procedure should not be performed on patients with active pelvic infections and antibiotic prophylaxis should be used in patients with a history of pelvic inflammatory disease[19].

Both doxycycline and metronidazole have been reported to be effective prophylactic agents. Color Doppler hysterosalpingography should be performed during the early follicular phase of the menstrual cycle, after complete cessation of menses. This avoids dispersion of menstrual debris into the peritoneal cavity. Procedures done in this period allow absorption of the media prior to ovulation, thus avoiding the presence of a foreign substance around the time of an imminent corpus luteum. This decreases any theoretic effect the media may have on tubal transport. Hysterosalpingography performed during the immediate premenstrual phase of the cycle has been advocated in the evolution of possible cervical incompetence, as that is the point in the cycle at which there is maximum uterine constric-

tion. Therefore, in order to maximize the information obtained, the indication for the study has an influence on timing.

Patients are informed of the benefits and the possible risks of the procedure and the procedure itself is described to them in detail. Premedication or sedation is routinely used: 5–10 mg of diazepam intravenously is beneficial, especially in anxious patients. Pain signifies the obstruction and potential intravasation or tubal rupture, and should not be masked by anesthesia.

The patient voids and is positioned supine on the gynecological table. With the patient's legs flexed, a speculum is inserted into the vagina and positioned such that the entire cervix is visualized and the os is easily accessible. The cervix and vagina are then thoroughly scrubbed with Betadine solution. A tenaculum is placed on the anterior lip of the cervix, and the cannula is gently guided into the endocervical canal.

Equipment needed to perform color Doppler hysterosalpingography includes an ultrasound unit with color Doppler capability and an intrauterine catheter[19]. The first observation to be made is of the uterine cavity, with verification of the catheter placement. After removal of the tenaculum, the transvaginal probe is gently introduced into the posterior fornix of the vagina. The contrast (sterile saline) is then injected slowly, under control of the ultrasound picture. Usually, no more then 5–10 ml of contrast is instilled into the uterine cavity. At this stage one can observe the morphology of the uterus and its endometrial lining and detect duplication anomalies of the uterus (Color plate 23) or existence of endometrial polyps (Figure 1; Color plate 24) or submucous fibroids (Figure 2; Color plate 25) that are protruding into the uterine cavity which is marked with anechoic contrast (Color plate 26). After that, the color Doppler observation is directed at the cornual region where the tubal catheter with a metal end should be located (Figure 3). The exact placement of the catheter is sonographically controlled. Color signals passing through the Fallopian tube indicate its patency (Color plate 27), while the absence of such signals is interpreted as tubal occlusion[20,21]. Accumulation of the fluid in the cul-de-sac on the side of injection controlled by transvaginal color and pulsed Doppler is an accurate indicator of

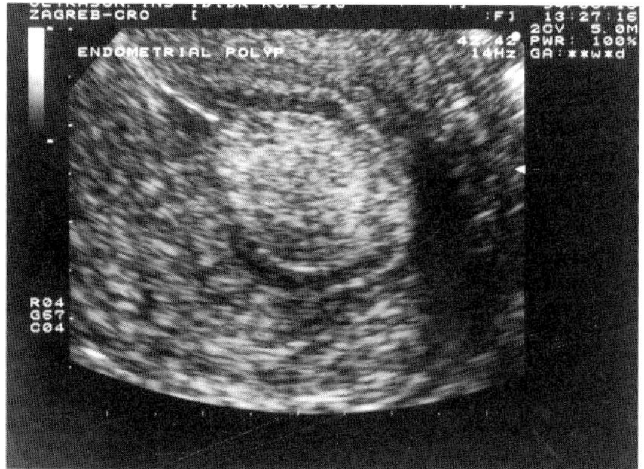

Figure 1 Transvaginal scan in a patient of reproductive age showing a focal polyp outlined by a small amount of injected saline solution

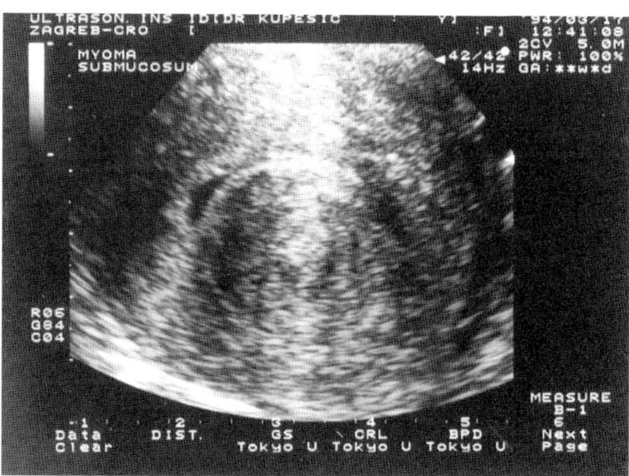

Figure 2 Transverse scan demonstrating submucous fibroid outlined by injection of a small amount of isotonic saline solution

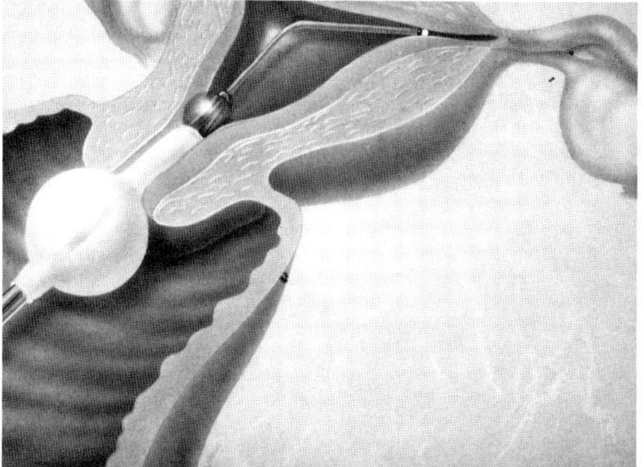

Figure 3 The intrauterine cannula (Bard) is placed into the uterus. Note two balloons: one is placed on the level of the internal cervical os, while another one is fixed in the external cervical os. A tiny tubal catheter with a metal end is introduced after the exploration of the uterine cavity

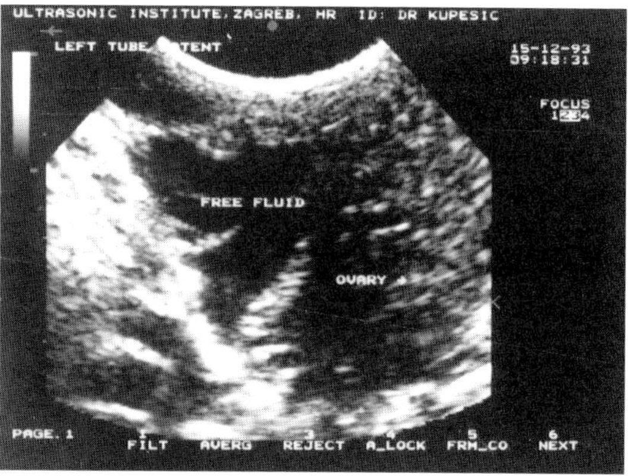

Figure 4 The same patient as in Color plate 27. Note anechoic contrast in the cul-de-sac after passage through the right Fallopian tube. Peritubal adhesions are visualized as thin and rigid connections within the pelvis

ipsilateral tubal pregnancy (Figure 4; Color plate 28). Undoubtedly, selective tubal injection increases the accuracy of the procedure and appropriateness of the interpretation. The procedure is repeated for the contralateral side (Color plate 29). If the patient complains of cramping during the procedure, the injection of saline should be stopped for a few minutes. Non-visualization of both tubes suggests cornual obstruction, but can represent spasm as well. Pretreatment with atropine (0.5 mg) may prevent this complication. The parenteral administration of 1 mg glucagon may relieve the spasm and allow the flow of the contrast[10,22,23].

Difficulty in making the diagnosis of tubal occlusion arises in those patients with dilated hydrosalpinges because flow through the dilated Fallopian tube may simulate spillage on the Doppler ultrasonography screen (Figure 5; Color plates 30 and 31). To avoid possible errors, we should perform careful observation of both adnexa before the procedure (Figure 6; Color plate 32). In addition, the tubal architecture is not demonstrated with Doppler flow hysterosalpingography. However, a recent study has shown this information not to be useful in preoperative salpingoplasty procedures[24].

Using our modified technique, we compared

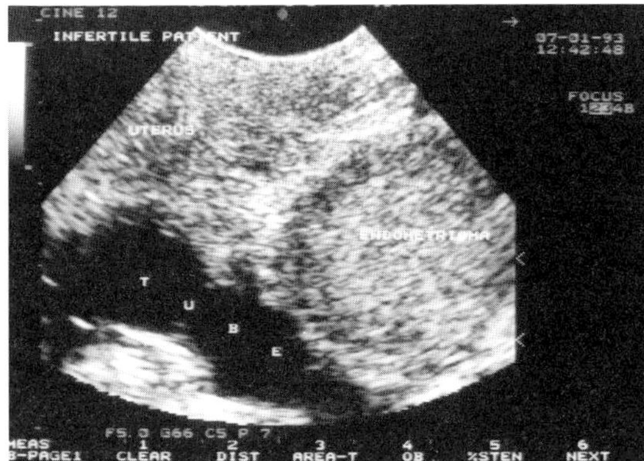

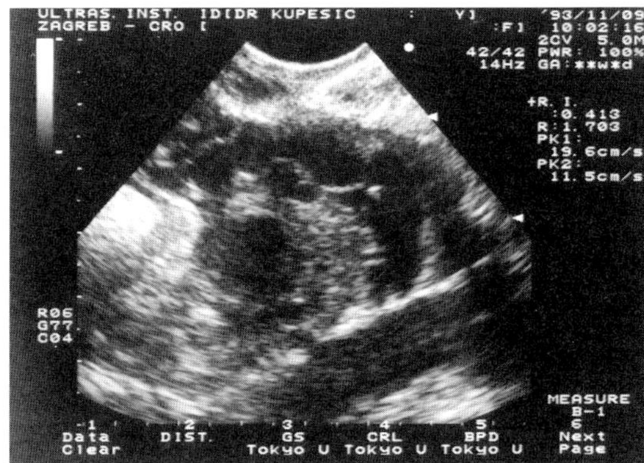

Figure 5 Transvaginal sonogram of a primary infertile patient undergoing color Doppler hysterosalpingography. Note the uniformly echogenic thick blood contents of the large endometriotic cyst. The ipsilateral tube is shown in the longitudinal section after the injection of isotonic saline. This finding indicates distal tubal occlusion

Figure 6 Complex adnexal mass that can be interpreted as a dilated tube surrounding the ovary

Table 2 Comparison of transvaginal color Doppler and hysterosalpingography (HSG) laparoscopic findings

	Bilateral patency	*Bilateral occlusion*	*Unilateral patency*
Transvaginal color Doppler HSG	23	12	12
Chromopertubation	24	10	13

the findings of color Doppler hysterosalpingography from 47 patients with those of chromopertubation at the time of laparoscopy[18]. The machines used were Aloka SSD 680 and 2000. Forty-three out of 47 (91.48%) color Doppler hysterosalpingography findings agreed with observations at chromopertubation (Table 2). In only one patient, in whom no patency was seen in both tubes under color Doppler evaluation, indirect diagnosis of tubal pregnancy was performed observing free fluid in the cul-de-sac.

Our results showed that transvaginal color Doppler hysterosalpingography is a safe and efficacious method for evaluation of Fallopian tube patency without exposure to radiation or contrast dyes. The cost of the procedure is significantly lower than for X-ray hysterosalpingography and it gives immediate results[10]. It is advisable that all the scans are recorded on video-recorder and/or Polaroid films[12] (Table 1).

Although the diagnostic usefulness of this method is unquestioned, one can speculate on the possible therapeutic action of the same modality[19]. The increased incidence of conception during the 3 months after the procedure (in our study, two patients) may be an effect of a mechanical lavage of the uterus by dislodging the mucous plugs, breakdown of the peritoneal adhesions, or a stimulatory effect on the tubal cilia.

No serious side-effects were observed during and after the transvaginal color Doppler hysterosalpingography procedure. Eighteen patients complained of pain that continued for 2–10 minutes after the procedure. No medication was required for these cases. The shortest time taken for the transvaginal color Doppler hysterosalpingography was 5 minutes, while the longest was 14 minutes. At the conclusion of the procedure, the speculum is repositioned and the instruments are removed. The cervix is inspected for hemostasis and pressure is applied to the tenaculum site whenever necessary.

To assess the accuracy of the diagnosis of tubal occlusion with the use of color Doppler flow ultra-

Table 3 The accuracy of ultrasound hysterosalpingography compared to X-ray hysterosalpingography

Reference	Total number	Accuracy (%)	Sensitivity	Specificity
Richman *et al.* (1984)[10]	36		100%	96%
Peters and Coulam (1991)[20]	27	19 (70.37)		
Volpi *et al.* (1991)[29]	21	19 (92.20)		
Stern *et al* (1992)[25]	89	72 (80.90)		

Table 4 The accuracy of ultrasound hysterosalpingography compared to chromopertubation

Reference	Total number	Accuracy (%)
Peters and Coulam (1991)[20]	58	50 (86.2)
Volpi *et al.* (1991)[29]	21	17 (83.3)
Tüfekci *et al.* (1992)[14]	38	37 (97.4)
Stern *et al.* (1992)[25]	121	99 (81.8)
Deichert *et al.* (1992)[26]	16	16 (100.0)
Allahbadia (1993)[8]	27	25 (92.6)
Kupesic and Kurjak (1994)[18]	47	43 (91.5)

sonography and hysterosalpingography, Peters and Coulam[20] studied 129 infertile women. Eighty-five of the 129 women also had an additional study including X-ray hysterosalpingography (Table 3) and/or chromopertubation (Table 4). Of these 85 women, 58 had pelviscopic examination with chromopertubation. The frequency of diagnosis of tubal occlusion was compared among the three methods. When results of ultrasonography–hysterosalpingography were compared with those of X-ray hysterosalpingography and/or chromopertubation, 69 of 85 (81%) studies showed agreement, and 50 out of 58 (86%) ultrasound hysterosalpingography findings agreed with observations at chromopertubation. The frequency of comparable findings between X-ray hysterosalpingography and chromopertubation is 75%.

Richman and colleagues[10] evaluated tubal patency in 36 infertile women. They compared ultrasound findings with conventional hysterosalpingograms, which had been obtained simultaneously. Ultrasound demonstrated bilateral occlusion with a sensitivity of 100%, and showed tubal patency with a specificity of 96% (Table 3).

Tüfekci and colleagues[14] studied 38 women with infertility complaints. The results obtained from transvaginal sonosalpingography and laparoscopy were completely consistent for 29 cases (76.32%), and partially consistent for eight cases (21.05%). Only one case (2.63%) showed an inconsistent result. Transvaginal sonosalpingography indicates tubal patency or non-patency in 37 of 38 cases (Table 4). When transvaginal sonosalpingography data are compared with laparoscopy, complete consistence means that the passage through both Fallopian tubes is identical by both methods. Partial consistence indicates identical results for only either the left or the right tube.

Stern and colleagues[25] administered saline transcervically during transvaginal color Doppler sonography in 238 women. Traditional X-ray hysterosalpingography was performed in 89 women. Laparoscopy with chromopertubation was performed in 121 women (Tables 3 and 4). Forty-nine women had all three procedures performed. Correlation between color ultrasound hysterosalpingography and X-ray findings with chromopertubation occurred in 81% versus 60% ($p = 0.0008$) of all women studied. In 49 women who had all three procedures performed, color ultrasound hysterosalpingography results correlated with chromopertubation more often than X-ray hysterosalpingography (82% versus 57%, $p = 0.0152$). In their previous report[20], discrepancies between color ultrasound hysterosalpingography and chromopertubation findings involved a diagnosis of unilateral patency. They recommend repeating color ultrasound hysterosalpingography before making a diagnosis of unilateral occlusion.

Deichert and colleagues[26] tried to determine whether the additional use of pulsed wave Doppler can improve the tubal diagnosis reached with gray-scale imaging in doubtful cases. They studied 17 patients with diagnosed sterility problems. Hysterosalpingo-contrast sonography by gray-scale and by pulsed wave Doppler and follow-up chromolaparoscopy ($n = 16$) (Table 4) or hysterosalpingography ($n = 1$) were performed. The diagnostic efficacies of gray scale and pulsed wave Doppler were compared with each other and with a conventional control procedure (chromolaparoscopy or hysterosalpingography).

The gray-scale findings were confirmed by pulsed wave Doppler in five cases on one side; confirmed by pulsed wave Doppler in seven cases on both sides; corrected by pulsed wave Doppler in four cases on one side; and corrected by pulsed wave Doppler in one case on one side and confirmed on the other side by pulsed wave Doppler. In all 17 cases, the tubal findings after pulsed wave Doppler were confirmed by chromolaparoscopy or hysterosalpingography. The additional use of pulsed wave Doppler in hysterosalpingo-contrast sonography is recommended as a supplement to gray-scale imaging in cases of suspected tubal occlusion and in the event of intratubal flow demonstrable only over a short distance.

Allahbadia[8] reported a 92.6% agreement between color Doppler ultrasonography compared with hysterosalpingography and laparoscopy. The hysterosalpingography and laparoscopy findings were in 100% agreement. The same author also described the so-called Sion procedure or hydrogynecography[27]. This procedure takes about 15 minutes as compared to the 5–6 minutes for sonosalpingography. After accomplishing sonosalpingography, sterile normal saline is injected until approximately 350 ml have flooded the pelvis. With the adnexa and uterus submerged in a fluid medium, the rescanning of the pelvis is repeated. If there is a bilateral tubal block and reflux of the saline is seen in the stem of the Foley's catheter, filling up the pelvis by alter-

native means is applied. The saline fills up the pelvis and delineates all sorts of adhesions; filmy and dense and even multiple thick septa in the periadnexal regions are depicted clearly. All the patients undergoing this procedure are similarly given prophylactic antibotics. The most frequent side-effect is significant cramping that patients feel as the fluid is injected through the cervix into the uterine cavity and through the Fallopian tubes. This can be minimized by injecting the fluid slowly or can be avoided by injecting the fluid directly into the cul-de-sac as done with bilaterally blocked tubes.

False-positive rates in the range of 9% and false-negative rates in the range of 20% have been reported in the diagnosis of tubal obstruction by color Doppler hysterosalpingography[25]. Therefore, all abnormal hysterosalpingogram studies deserve laparoscopic or hysteroscopic follow-up.

Normal X-ray or color Doppler hysterosalpingography does not rule out the need for diagnostic laparoscopy. Substantial criticism has been raised by some authors concerning the cost and some aspects of diagnostic efficacy of this method. Statistically founded studies comparing the cost of ultrasonography to X-ray hysterosalpingography are lacking. In such comparisons the cost of an ultrasonographic machine with color Doppler capability, coupled with indirect cost (equipment depreciation and physician time) should be considered. Balen and colleagues[28] found ultrasound contrast hysterosalpingography using both negative (sterile saline) and positive (Echovist) contrast media to be insufficiently accurate and inferior to conventional X-ray hysterosalpingography in the determination of tubal patency.

While X-ray hysterosalpingography is the most accurate method of diagnosing intramural or intraluminal abnormalities of the Fallopian tube, color Doppler hysterosalpingography is the only available non-invasive method for analyzing tubal motility. Thus, it is possible to obtain a significant amount of information from a properly performed ultrasound hysterosalpingogram (Table 1).

The most accurate interpretation can be obtained during the procedure itself, as the course of the medium is followed throughout the reproductive tract. Therefore, to obtain maximum information, the procedure should be performed by a well-trained physician who is familiar with the color Doppler investigation, and who is capable of manipulating the instruments, the patient's reproductive tract, and the rate of injection.

References

1. Hill, M.L. (1992). Infertility and reproductive assistance. In Neiberg, D.A., Hill, L.M., Bohm-Velez, M. and Mendelson, E.B. (eds.) *Transvaginal Ultrasound*, pp.43–6. (St. Louis: Mosby Year Book)

2. Arronet, G.M., Aduljie, S.Y. and O'Brien, I.R. (1969). A 9 year survey of Fallopian tube dysfunction in human infertility: diagnosis and therapy. *Fertil. Steril.*, **20**, 903–18

3. Rubin, I. (1954). Differences between the uterus and tubes as a cause of oscillations recorded during uterotubal insufflation. *Fertil. Steril.*, **5**, 147–53

4. Page, H. (1989). Estimation of the prevalence and incidence of infertility in a population: a pilot study. *Fertil. Steril.*, **71**, 571–4

5. McRac, M.E. (1988). Hysterosalpingography. In Garcia, C.R., Mastroianni, L., Amelar, R.D. and Dubin, L. (eds.) *Current Therapy of Infertility*, pp.1–3. (Toronto: BC Decker Inc)

6. Kerin, J.F., Williams, D.B., San Roman, G.A., Pearistone, A.C., Grundfest, W.S. and Sucrey, E.S. (1992). Falloposcopic classification and treatment of Fallopian tube disease. *Fertil. Steril.*, **57**, 731–5

7. Thurmond, A.S. and Rosch, J. (1990). Non-surgical Fallopian tube recanalization for treatment of infertility. *Radiology*, **174**, 371–4

8. Allahbadia, G.N. (1993). Fallopian tube patency using color Doppler. *Int. J. Gynecol. Obstet.*, **40**, 241–4

9. Timor-Tritsch, I.E. and Rottem, S. (1987). Transvaginal ultrasonographic study of the Fallopian tube. *Obstet. Gynecol.*, **70**, 424–8

10. Richman, T.S., Bisconi, G.N., de Cherney, A., Polan, M.L. and Alcebo, L.O. (1984). Fallopian tubal patency assessed by ultrasound following fluid injection. *Radiology*, **152**, 502–4

11. Randolph, J.R., Ying, Y.K., Maier, D.B., Scmidt, C.L. and Ridelick, D.H. (1986). Comparison of real time ultrasonography, laparoscopy and hysteroscopy in the evaluation of uterine abnormalities and tubal patency. *Fertil. Steril.*, **46**, 828–30

12. Deichert, U., Schlief, R., van de Sandt, M. and Junke, I. (1989). Transvaginal hysterosalpingo-contrast sonography (Hy-Co-Sy) compared with conventional tubal diagnostics. *Hum. Reprod.*, **4**, 418–22

13. Deichert, U., Schlief, R., van de Sandt, M., Goebel, R. and Daume, E. (1990). Transvaginale Hysterosalpingo-Kontrastosonographie (HKSG) im B-Bild Verfahren und in der farbcodierten Dublexsonographie zur Abklaerung der Tubenpassage. *Geburtshilfe Frauenheilkd.*, **50**, 717–22

14. Tüfekci, E.C., Girit, S., Bayirli, M.D., Durmusoglu, F. and Yalti, S. (1992). Evaluation of tubal patency by transvaginal sonosalpingography. *Fertil. Steril.*, **57**, 336–40

15. Gramiak, R. and Shah, P.M. (1968). Echocardiography of the aortic root. *Invest. Radiol.*, **3**, 356–66

16. Meltzer, R.S., Tickner, G., Sahines, T.P. and Popp, R.L. (1980). The source of ultrasound contrast effect. *J. Clin. Ultrasound*, **8**, 121

17. Suren, A., Puchta, J. and Osmers, R. (1995). Fluid instillation into the uterine cavity. In Osmers, R. and Kurjak, A. (eds.) *Ultrasound and The Uterus*, pp. 45–51. (Carnforth, UK: Parthenon Publishing)

18. Kupesic, S. and Kurjak, A. (1994). Gynecological vaginal sonographic interventional procedures – what does color add? *Gynecol. Perinatol.*, **3**, 57–60

19. Kupesic, S. and Kurjak, A. (1994). The role of color Doppler in vaginal sonographic puncture procedures. In Kurjak, A. (ed.) *An Atlas of Transvaginal Color Doppler*, pp.335–47. (Carnforth, UK: Parthenon Publishing)

20. Peters, J.A. and Coulam, C.B. (1991). Hysterosalpingography with color Doppler ultrasonography. *Am. J. Obstet. Gynecol.*, **164**, 1530–2

21. Peters, J.A., Stern, J.J. and Coulam, C.B. (1992). Color Doppler hysterosalpingography. In Jaffe, R. and Warsof, S.L. (eds.) *Color Doppler in Obstetrics and Gynecology*, p.283. (New York: McGraw Hill)

22. McCalley, M., Braunstein, P., Stone, S., Henderson, P. and Egbeat, R. (1985). Radionuclide hysterosalpingography for evaluation of Fallopian tube pregnancy. *J. Nucl. Med.*, **26**, 868–70

23. Keirse, M. and Wunderwellen, R. (1973). A comparison of hysterosalpingography and laparoscopy in the investigation of infertility. *Obstet. Gynecol.*, **41**, 685–8

24. Groff, T.R., Edelstein, J.A. and Schenken, R.S. (1990). Hysterosalpingography in the preoperative evaluation of tubal anastomosis candidates. *Fertil. Steril.*, **53**, 417–20

25. Stern, J., Peters, A.J. and Coulam, C.B. (1992). Color Doppler ultrasonography assessment of tubal patency: a comparison study with traditional technique. *Fertil. Steril.*, **58**, 897–900

26. Deichert, U., Schlief, R., van de Sandt, M. and Daume, E. (1992). Transvaginal hysterosalpingo-contrast sonography for the assessment of tubal patency with grey-scale imaging and additional use of pulsed wave Doppler. *Fertil. Steril.*, **57**, 62–7

27. Allahbadia, G., Nalawade, Y., Panjwani, M., Vaydia, P. and Merchant, S. (1992). The Sion procedure. *J. Obstet. Gynecol. India*, **42**, 814–18

28. Balen, F.G., Allen, C.M., Siddle, N.C. and Lees, W.R. (1993). Ultrasound contrast hysterosalpingography – evaluation as an outpatient procedure. *Br. J. Radiol.*, **66**, 592–9

29. Volpi, E., De Grandis, T., Sismondi, P., Giacardi, M., Rustichelli, S., Patriarca, A. and Bocci, A. (1991). Transvaginal salpingo-sonography (TSSG) in the evaluation of tubal patency. *Acta Eur. Fertil.*, **22**, 325–8

Index